UCL
Hospitals
Injectable Drug Administration Guide

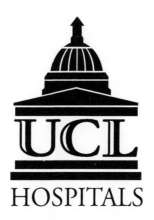

Injectable Drug Administration Guide

Edited by

Robert Shulman, Sarla Drayan, Mark Harries, Denise Hoare and Simon Badcott

The Pharmacy Department,
University College London Hospitals

Blackwell
Science

Blackwell Science Ltd, a Blackwell Publishing Company
Editorial Offices:
Blackwell Science Ltd, 9600 Garsington Road, Oxford OX4 2DQ, UK
    Tel: +44 (0) 1865 776868
Blackwell Publishing Inc., 350 Main Street, Malden, MA 02148-5020, USA
    Tel: +1 781 388 8250
Blackwell Science Asia Pty, 550 Swanston Street, Carlton, Victoria 3053, Australia
    Tel: +61 (0) 3 8359 1011

First published 1998
Reprinted 2000, 2002, 2003, 2004

ISBN 0-632-05027-6

A catalogue record for this title is available from the British Library

Printed and bound in India by Replika Press Pvt. Ltd.

The publisher's policy is to use permanent paper from mills that operate a sustainable forestry policy, and which has been manufactured from pulp processed using acid-free and elementary chlorine-free practices. Furthermore, the publisher ensures that the text paper and cover board used have met acceptable environmental accreditation standards.

For further information on Blackwell Publishing, visit our website:
www.blackwellpublishing.com

CONTENTS

ACKNOWLEDGEMENTS

The *UCL Hospitals Injectable Drug Administration Guide* is the result of an extensive team effort, some members of which have changed since the book was published within UCL Hospitals.

We would like to thank the listed contributors and to extend our thanks to other groups who provided helpful comments including the UCL Hospitals Nursing Practice Committee particularly Michael Flynn and Tim Jackson.

We would also like to recognise the contribution of the Pharmacy Department of the Hammersmith Hospital and to Susan Keeling and the pharmacists who have contributed to The IV Guide.

Finally our thanks to Richard Miles at Blackwell Science Ltd for his encouragement and patience.

Sarla Drayan   **Robert Shulman**
Clinical Pharmacy Services manager   **Formulary Pharmacist**

CONTRIBUTORS

Simon Badcott, *MRPharmS, Dip Clin Pharm*
Intensive Care Pharmacist

Jeff Bradley, *MRPharmS*
Production Specialist Pharmacist

Sarah Bull,
formerly UCLH Pre-registration Pharmacist

Liam Carter, *MRPharmS, Dip Clin Pharm*
Imaging and Cardiac Pharmacist

Jane Davey, *MRPharmS, Cert Clin Pharm*
formerly UCLH Pharmacist

Alex Fotherby, *MRPharmS, Cert Clin Pharm*
formerly UCLH Pharmacist

Chris Hampton, *MRPharmS*
Dispensary Manager

Mark Harries, *MRPharmS, MSc*
Paediatrics, Acute Pain Pharmacist

Rachel Heylen, *MRPharmS, MSc*
HIV/AIDs Pharmacist

Sue Imison, *MRPharmS, ADCPT*
Education & Training Pharmacist

Deirdre Linnard, *MRPharmS, Dip Clin Pharm*
Surgery and Gasteroenterology, Acute Pain Pharmacist

Shameem Mir, *MRPharmS, Dip Clin Pharm*
formerly UCLH Mental Health Pharmacist

Anu Paul, *MRPharmS, Cert Clin Pharm*
Women's Services Pharmacist

Jane Ratcliffe, *MRPharmS, Dip Clin Pharm*
Theatres and Musculo-skeletal Pharmacist

Robert Shulman, *MRPharmS, Dip Clin Pharm*
Formulary Pharmacist

Rachel Tebay, *MRPharmS, Cert Clin Pharm*
formerly UCLH Pharmacist

Cathy Beer, *MRPharmS, Dip Clin Pharm*
Haematology Pharmacist

Tracey Brown, *MRPharmS, Dip Clin Pharm*
Urology & Nephrology, Acute Pain Pharmacist

Dorwin Cardozo, *MPharmS, Cert Clin Pharm*
General Medicine Pharmacist

Zareena Davar, *MRPharmS, Cert Clin Pharm*
formerly UCLH Pharmacist

Sarla Drayan, *MRPharmS, MCPP, MSc, MBA*
Clinical Pharmacy Services Manager

Paul Grayston, *MRPharmS, Cert Clin Pharm*
Production Pharmacist

Rabiha Hannan,
formerly UCLH Pre-registration Pharmacist

Richard Healey, *BSc, MSc*
Medical Physics Technical Officer

Denise Hoare, *MRPharmS, MSc*
Oncology Pharmacist

Anna Lam, *MRPharmS, Cert Clin Pharm*
Drug Information & Clinical Trials Pharmacist

Russell Mills, *MRPharmS, Dip Clin Pharm*
formerly Dispensary Pharmacist

Tony Murphy, *MRPharmS, MSc*
Production Services Pharmacist

June Randall, *MRPharmS, Dip Clin Pharm*
HIV/AIDs Support Pharmacist

Christine Richardson, *MRPharmS, Dip Clin Pharm*
General Medicine Pharmacist

Sharon Steele, *MRPharmS, Cert Clin Pharm*
Community Services Pharmacist

viii

1. INTRODUCTION

The use of injectable drugs is part of everyday practice in hospitals and increasingly so in primary care. The relevant information needed for administration is often not easily accessible. With this consideration in mind we decided to develop a single reference source for this information at UCLH.

Although some hospitals have their own *intravenous* drug administration guides, the *UCL Hospitals Injectable Drug Administration Guide* includes routes other than the IV route. It also incorporates some policies and guidances which we hope will be invaluable reference points as they are expanded.

The *UCLH Injectable Drug Administration Guide* seeks to provide an easy to use reference source of information and advice on the administration of drugs given by the injectable route (intravenously, intramuscularly, subcutaneously). The guide is intended to help doctors, nurses, pharmacists and other health professionals with an interest and involvement in injectable drugs.

☞ 2.1 ORGANISATION OF INFORMATION IN THE GUIDE

There are two sections in the *UCL Hospitals Injectable Drug Administration Guide.*

Section A includes general information: explanatory notes on the abbreviations used and the type of information included, the responsibility of different professional groups, preparation on wards, guidance on flushing lines and cannulae, infusion pumps, discharge information, management of extravasation, syringe pump compatibility and pharmaceutical aspects of intravenous therapy.

Section B contains the individual drug details on 210 drugs in a tabular form. Drugs are arranged in alphabetical order and the following information is included :-

- formulation
- injectable method of administration
- preparation of the drug
- administration details
- stability
- compatibility
- pH
- flush
- sodium content
- displacement value
- acute bedside monitoring

It does not include information on cytotoxic drugs or those solely administered by the intramuscular or subcutaneous route.

☛ 2.2 SOURCES OF INFORMATION

The information and advice in the *UCL Hospitals Injectable Drug Administration Guide* is based on the best available published data at the time of going to print. Note however that published compatibility data is ***not*** available for all the combinations and situations covered in this guide. Some of the advice and information therefore reflects local practice and experience only. In addition readers are reminded that slight variation in the exact combination and concentrations of drugs can adversely affect compatibility. Readers are referred to their local hospital pharmacy department for more specific information and advice. Neither the authors nor the publisher can accept any legal responsibility or liability for any errors or omission which may be made. Readers should take their own precautions to ensure that new information after the book was written is followed wherever possible. Readers are referred to the 'summary of product characteristics' (data sheets) produced by the pharmaceutical companies. These are periodically updated and thus the recommendation(s) for administering the medicines included in this guide may alter from time to time.

☛ 2.3 UPDATES AND THE NEXT EDITION

Time has not allowed us to cover all the many aspects involved in the subject of injectable drug administration in this edition. It is intended to continually improve future editions. Possible examples for improvement include expansion of the introductory section to provide a more comprehensive reference source including information that is useful across the healthcare sectors and to reference the sources of information.

Your comments, criticisms, suggestions for improvement, advice on changes will be gratefully received. This feedback is essential to ensure the *UCL Hospitals Injectable Drug Administration Guide* continues to be an accurate, useful, current, comprehensive and easy to use source of information.

Please send your comments to:

Robert Shulman	or	Sarla Drayan
Formulary Pharmacist UCLH		Clinical Pharmacy Services Manager
Pharmacy Department		
Middlesex Hospital		
Mortimer Street		
London		
W1N 8AA		

☞ 2.4 ABBREVIATIONS USED IN THIS GUIDE

2.4.1 Methods of administration

Abbreviation	Method of administration	Definition/description
(C) IV infusion	Continuous intravenous infusion	Intravenous administration of a volume of fluid with or without drugs added over 24 hours or over a number of hours to achieve a given clinical endpoint. The infusion may be repeated over a period of days. Large volume i.e. 250 - 1,000ml or small volume infusions (e.g. 50ml of heparin) may be delivered continuously.
(I) IV infusion	Intermittent intravenous infusion	Administration of an infusion over a set time period, either as a one-off dose or repeated at specific time intervals.
IV bolus	Intravenous bolus	Introduction of a small volume of drug solution into the cannula or the injection site of an administration set. A bolus injection should be administered over 3 - 5 minutes unless otherwise specified.
S/C	Subcutaneous injection	
(C) S/C infusion	Continuous subcutaneous infusion	
IM	Intramuscular injection	

2.4.2 Fluids

Abbreviation	Fluid
N/S	Sodium chloride 0.9% BP (normal saline)
G	Glucose 5% BP
W	Water for injection (preservative free) BP
G/S	Glucose 4% and sodium chloride 0.18% BP
H	Compound sodium lactate (Hartmann's)
Hep/S	Heparin 10units in 1ml sodium chloride 0.9% - heparinised sodium chloride (e.g. Hepsal, Heplok)

☛ 2.5 'ACUTE EVENTS WHICH MAY ACCOMPANY ADMINISTRATION'

Acute events which may accompany administration have been detailed where possible to warn the nurse or doctor administering the drug of the most common adverse effects which may occur at the time or immediately after administration. The events listed are not comprehensive and do not cover delayed side effects or those which cannot be monitored at the bedside.

☛ 2.6 INTRAVENOUS DRUG COMPATIBILITY INFORMATION

Since the information available is limited, drugs should ideally be infused separately.

The drug compatibility section in the administration table contains information which is mainly based on physical compatibility, i.e. no visible sign of incompatibility after 4 hours. When two drugs are described as Y-site compatible it is assumed that standard concentrations of both drugs are being mixed in a line and not in an infusion bag, burette or syringe. The compatibility information is not definitive, since varying the drug concentration may produce signs of incompatibility (e.g. cloudiness, change in colour, haze or precipitation). This section has been left blank where there is no useful compatibility information available at the time of going to print. The drugs included in the compatibility section are not comprehensive and refer only to likely combinations of drugs used in UCL Hospitals.

Where two drugs are infused simultaneously via a Y-site, the distal portion of the line should be examined for signs of incompatibility.

When using the compatibility information, ensure that both drugs are compatible with the infusion fluids in use.

Readers are referred to their local hospital pharmacy department regarding drug compatibility combinations that are not addressed in this guide and for further information on a given combination.

☛ 2.7 pH VALUES

2.7.1 Incompatibility

pH values are included to help predict possible physical incompatibility among drugs where no compatibility information exists. It is not advisable to simultaneously administer drugs with widely differing pH values as this may result in incompatibility leading to precipitation or inactivation of either or both drugs.

2.7.2 Irritancy

pH values are also used to indicate the irritancy of a drug, see section 7.2.4 for full details.

☛ 2.8 DISPLACEMENT VALUES

Where the dose of a drug is less than a complete vial and the vial requires reconstitution e.g. for paediatrics, it is necessary to take into account the displacement value of the drug.

For example: To give a dose of 125mg amoxycillin from a 250mg vial.
The displacement value of amoxycillin 250mg is 0.2ml.
If 4.8ml of diluent is added to a 250mg vial, the volume of the resulting solution is 5ml (i.e. 4.8ml + 0.2ml).
Therefore 125mg will be contained in 2.5ml of the solution.

☞3.1 RESPONSIBILITIES OF PROFESSIONAL STAFF AT UCLH

3.1.1 Nurses' Responsibilities For Injectable Drugs
(including Blood Products, IV Fluids and IV Drugs)

Nurses are referred to the 'Standards for the Administration of Medicines', United Kingdom Central Council for Nursing, Midwifery and Health Visitors.

At UCL Hospitals, injectable drugs may be prepared and administered by a registered nurse /midwife as described in UCL Hospitals 'Administration of Medicines by Nurses/ Midwives Policy and Procedure' document. This document is available from UCL Hospitals.

3.1.2 Pharmacists' Responsibilities For Injectable Drugs

❑ Pharmacists monitor prescriptions for parenteral drugs and alert medical and/or nursing staff to any potential problems. Pharmacists should annotate prescriptions for parenteral drugs where appropriate.
❑ Pharmacists should provide appropriate information and advice to medical, nursing and other health professionals on all the pharmaceutical aspects of parenteral drugs e.g. choice of drug therapy, compatibility, stability, dosage, administration details.
❑ Pharmacists provide education and training to health professionals involved in the administration of parenteral medicines.
❑ Pharmacy will prepare complex drugs to be administered by the parenteral route as locally agreed.

☞3.2 PREPARATION OF INJECTABLE DRUGS ON WARDS, CLINICS AND DEPARTMENTS AT UCLH

Injectable drugs:
❑ **Must not** be prepared in advance of their immediate use.
❑ **Must not** be prepared by anyone other than the registered nurse/ midwife or doctor who is going to administer them, unless they are prepared in his/her presence.

All drugs prepared must be appropriately labelled. Additive labels should be completed and attached to the infusion container.

Exceptions:

Injectable drugs may only be prepared in advance if covered by a specific protocol agreed by relevant pharmacy and nursing staff.

☞ 3.3 CHECKLIST FOR PREPARING AND ADMINISTERING INTRAVENOUS DRUGS

- ❏ Pre-plan before drawing up doses
- ❏ Be sure of local protocols
- ❏ Check drug against the prescription - check that the dose, time and route is correct
- ❏ Check patient identification
- ❏ Check IV site
- ❏ Check that any equipment required is working
- ❏ Know how to administer each drug
  - calculation of concentration and rate
  - reconstitution
  - addition of drugs to recommended diluents
  - check package insert, Data Sheet, UCL Hospitals Injectable Drug Administration Guide and Pharmacy Drug Information Centre for further information
- ❏ Use aseptic technique during reconstitution steps, addition of drug to diluents, and care of the line
- ❏ Maintain a sterile, particle-free solution
- ❏ Thoroughly mix any additions, checking for precipitation or particles
- ❏ Complete yellow infusion additive label and attach to infusion
- ❏ Understand how the drug works and explain this to the patient if appropriate
- ❏ Continue to monitor for precipitation and patient response where appropriate

IF IN DOUBT ASK / CHECK WITH A PHARMACIST, NURSING COLLEAGUE OR DOCTOR.

4. GUIDELINES ON FLUSHING LINES AND CANNULAE

☞ 4.1 FLUSHING BETWEEN DRUGS

Flushing between administration of individual drugs must be carried out to avoid interaction between incompatible drugs. Unless the drugs concerned are known to be compatible, flushing between drugs must be undertaken.

Cannulae: 5-10ml of either sodium chloride 0.9% (N/S) or glucose 5% (G) can be used for flushing. Check the individual drug monograph for details of which flushing solution to use.

Lines: Following drug administration via an infusion line, the line should be flushed by connecting a bag containing one of the compatible infusion fluids. This should be administered at a rate not exceeding that recommended for administration of the original drug. Approximately 20ml must be infused, preferably from a 500ml bag of sodium chloride 0.9% (N/S) or glucose 5% (G) which is cheaper than a 100ml bag.

☞ 4.2 FLUSHING CANNULAE NOT IN USE

Peripheral cannulae: Flush 5ml sodium chloride 0.9% (N/S) 8 hourly to maintain patency of peripheral cannulae where there is no continuous infusion, unless drugs are being administered through the cannula at 8 hourly intervals or more frequently.

Central lines: UCL Hospitals staff follow a locally produced skin tunnelled central line catheter policy.

Fatal errors have been reported following the incorrect administration of drugs via infusion pumps. It is the responsibility of the person administering the drug to ensure that an appropriate pump is being used, it is in good working order, and that they know how to operate it correctly. Alterations to the pump settings must be made by a person authorised to administer intravenous drugs. The volume of fluid administered should be recorded on the fluid chart. All pumps should be checked frequently during the infusion.

☛ 5.1 CHOICE OF PUMPS USED AT UCLH

5.1.1 Drip Rate Controller *(IVAC 231)*

The infusion rate is selected in drops per minute and the flow is gravity fed.

5.1.2 Volumetric Pumps *(IVAC 591, 598, 598; Baxter F2M8043E)*

These are the preferred pumps for medium and large volume infusions; although some are designed specifically to operate at low flow rates for neonatal use. The rate is selected in millilitres per hour (usual range 1 - 999ml per hour). Typically, most volumetric pumps are accurate to ± 5% at rates down to 5ml per hour. A syringe pump should be used for rates lower than 5ml per hour.

5.1.3 Syringe Pumps *(e.g. Graseby 3300, 9000, MS 2000, 3100, 3400; IVAC/Welmed P1000, P2000, 701; Vickers IP5)*

These are low volume, high accuracy devices designed to infuse low flow rates and are typically calibrated for delivery in millilitres per hour (usual range 0.1 - 99ml per hour). Many pumps will accept different sizes and different brands of syringe, but the pumps must be set up for the particular type and size of syringe in use, unless the pump detects the syringe size and type automatically. The Medicines Device Agency recommends rates below 0.5 ml per hour should not be used unless the pump is specially designed for this purpose, as an increase in the occlusion response time occurs.

5.1.4   <u>Pumps for Ambulatory Use</u>

i) Miniature syringe pumps (syringe drivers) *(Graseby MS16 blue, MS26 green)*

These pumps typically accept syringes between 2 and 10ml and are able to achieve very low flow rates of delivery. They may require the rate to be set in **millimetres** per **hour** or **millimetres** per **day** i.e. linear travel of syringe plunger against time. Calculations which depend on the syringe size used are required to convert from flow rate to linear travel per unit time.

ii) Miniature volumetric pumps *(Graseby 9100, 9300, Walkmed 350)*

These pumps use reservoirs which contain the solution within the pump. Some offer a variety of programming options.

5.1.5   <u>Patient Controlled Analgesia (PCA) Pumps</u>   *(Graseby 3300 PCA)*

They are typically syringe pumps, but have the facility to enable patients to administer a bolus dose to themselves. A PCA pump has several programming options which may be set by specified clinical staff. With PCA pumps, protection against free-flow is important, as the patient may be unsupervised for some of the time.

A different type of PCA device involves the use of an elastomeric reservoir (Baxter PCA) or syringe reservoir (Vygon PCA). Unlike electronic PCA pumps they have no programming features.

6. DISCHARGE INFORMATION FOR COMMUNITY NURSES INVOLVED IN THE ADMINISTRATION OF IV MEDICINES

Increasingly, patients are discharged on intravenous (IV) therapy for use at home. Often the task of intravenous administration falls on community nurses. Although community nurses may have access to their own IV administration policies and training, they work in isolation and may not be familiar with the IV drugs that they are asked to administer.

Community nurses may therefore require information and advice on the intravenous medicine(s) prior to visiting the patient at home. Some may wish to visit the patient on the ward prior to discharge, to familiarise themselves with the drug, the type of equipment and the skills required for care. The information required by the community nurse will include:

- ❏ Name of medication
- ❏ Indication for use
- ❏ Dose
- ❏ Patient weight/body surface area/clinical status (as appropriate)
- ❏ Method of administration
- ❏ For IV infusions-diluent and volume/concentrations/rate/duration of infusion
- ❏ Method of rate control
- ❏ Frequency of administration (Community nurse schedules and patient convenience may need consideration)
- ❏ Storage requirements
- ❏ Arrangements for ongoing prescription and supply of medicines
- ❏ Arrangements for disposal of clinical waste
- ❏ Side effects
- ❏ Clinically significant interactions
- ❏ Monitoring
- ❏ Reconstitution in the patient's home may pose additional training needs and COSHH (control of substances hazardous to health) implications must be considered

For licensed products the above information will usually be available from the B.N.F., data sheets and package inserts. Where medicines are prescribed outside of the recommendations of the product licence, community nurses require access to sufficient information to satisfy themselves that the prescription is appropriate in the context of the condition of the patient at the time of administration by the nurse. The necessary information should be made available at the time of discharge from the ward. Prescribing guidelines, shared care guidelines and pharmacy discharge plans are a useful source of information.

7. MANAGEMENT OF EXTRAVASATION OF INTRAVENOUS DRUGS

Extravasation is the accidental infiltration of intravenous fluids into the subcutaneous tissue. It can occur for a number of reasons and may lead to an inflammatory response and/or pain from the affected tissue which may be immediate or delayed. *The potential for a delayed reaction should be remembered when the initial assessment of a suspected extravasation site is made.*

It has been shown in several studies that a patient's risk of extravasation is dependent upon several factors.

☛ 7.1 PATIENT FACTORS AFFECTING EXTRAVASATION

Certain groups of patients are more likely to develop problems following extravasation; these include:

7.1.1 Neonates

Neonates possess much less subcutaneous tissue relative to an adult. Hence any extravasated material is more concentrated in the affected area. They are also much less able to accurately vocalise their pain (see below).

7.1.2 Patients Unable To Vocalise / Communicate Their Pain

Comatosed, anaesthetised patients and those being resuscitated are not able to provide clear vocalisation of the pain caused by the extravasation of a substance. They (and the neonates mentioned above) form perhaps the group of patients at greatest risk from extravasation.

7.1.3 Patients Unable To Sense Pain

Special care should also be taken when administering intravenous drugs to patients who have an impaired ability to detect pain. Patients who suffer from peripheral neuropathy (e.g. diabetics) are one such group.

☞ 7.2 DRUG FACTORS AFFECTING EXTRAVASATION

7.2.1 Cytotoxic Drugs

Several cytotoxic agents will cause extensive tissue damage if extravasated. Some of these agents require specific treatment when extravasation occurs; such advice is outside the scope of this guide.

7.2.2 Vasoconstrictor Drugs

When these drugs are administered peripherally, extravasation can produce local vasoconstriction leading to severe tissue hypoxia and ischaemia.

7.2.3 Irritant Drugs

The following factors need to be considered prior to giving an intravenous drug:

7.2.3. (i) pH

Solutions with a high or low pH will cause more tissue damage if they are extravasated. The table on the next page shows examples of drugs that have high or low pHs.

DRUGS WITH HIGH OR LOW pHs

Intravenous Injection	pH	Intravenous Injection	pH
Acetazolamide	9.2	Labetalol	3.5 - 4.2
Aciclovir	11	Lignocaine	3.5 - 6
Adrenaline	2.5 - 3.6	Liothyronine	11
Allopurinol	10.8 - 11. 8	Methohexitone	10 - 11
Aminophylline	8.8 - 10	Methoxamine	4.4
Amiodarone	3.5 - 4.5	Methyldopa	3 - 4.2
Anti-thymocyte immunoglobulin rabbit (ATG Fresenius)	3.7	Methylene blue	3 - 4.5
Argipressin	2.5 - 5.4	Metoclopramide	3 - 5
Atracurium	3.5	Midazolam	3
Atropine	3 - 6.5	Morphine	2.3 - 4.5
Azathioprine	10 - 12	Naloxone	3 - 4.5
Buprenorphine	3.5 - 5.5	Noradrenaline acid tartrate	3 - 4.5
Cholecystokinin (CCK)	3 - 6	Octreotide	3.9 - 4.5
Clonazepam	3.5 - 4.5	Omeprazole	9 - 10
Co-trimoxazole	9 - 10.5	Ondansetron	3.4 - 3.8
Cyclizine	3.3 - 3.7	Oxytocin	3.7 - 4.3
Dantrolene	9.5	Pancuronium	3.8 - 4.2
Diazoxide	11.6	Papaveretum	2.5 - 4
Dobutamine	3.5 - 4	Phenobarbitone	9 - 10.5
Dopamine	2.5 - 4.5	Phenoxybenzamine	2.5 - 3.1
Doxapram	3 - 5	Phenytoin sodium	12
Droperidol	2.7 - 4.7	Potassium canrenoate	10.7 - 11.2
Elohaes	3.5	Prochlorperazine	3.9 - 4.5
Epoprostenol	10.5	Procyclidine	3.9 - 4.5
Ergometrine	2.7 - 3.5	Propranolol	3
Fentanyl	3.3 - 6.3	Protamine sulphate	2.5 - 3.5
Folic acid	8 - 11	Quinine dihydrochloride	2 - 3
Frusemide	8.7 - 9.3	Salbutamol	3.5
Ganciclovir	10 - 11	Secretin	2.5 - 5
Gentamicin	3 - 5	Sodium nitroprusside	3.5 - 6
Glucagon	2.5 - 3	Sulphadiazine	11
Glucose (pH dependent on concentration of solution)	3.5 - 6.5	Terbutaline	3 - 5
Glyceryl trinitrate	3.5 - 6.5	Tetracosactrin	3.8 - 4.5
Glycopyrronium	2.3 - 4.3	Tetracycline	1.8
Haloperidol	3 - 3.8	Thiamine	2.5 - 4.5
Hydralazine	3.5 - 4.2	Thiopentone	10.5
Hyoscine butylbromide	3.7 - 5.5	Tobramycin	3.5 - 6
Isoprenaline	2.5 - 2.8	Tubocurarine	3.8 - 4
Ketamine	3.5 - 5.5	Vancomycin	2.8 - 4.5

This is not a comprehensive list.

7.2.3. (ii) Osmolarity

Solutions with an osmolarity greater than that of plasma (>290mOsmol/l) may cause tissue damage. The presence of these solutions can lead to an osmotic imbalance across the cell membrane, a breakdown of the cellular transport mechanisms and cell death. The majority of intravenous drugs are formulated to have equal osmotic pressure as plasma so that the solution to be injected into the patient is unlikely to cause disturbance to the tissues. The table below lists a selection of the drugs included in the *UCL Hospitals Injectable Drug Administration Guide* that have high osmolarity and may potentially cause a problem if extravasated. Extra care should be taken when administering these drugs.

DRUGS WITH HIGH OSMOLARITY

Intravenous Injection	Osmolarity (mOsmol/L)	Intravenous Injection	Osmolarity (mOsmol/L)
Glucose 10%	535	Mannitol 10%	550
Glucose 20%	1,110	Mannitol 20%	1,100
Glucose 50%	2,775	Magnesium sulphate 50%	4,060
Calcium Gluconate 10%	670	Potassium chloride 20mmol/10ml	4,000
Calcium Chloride 5 mmol/10ml	1,500	Sodium bicarbonate 4.2%	1,004
Diazepam (CP Pharmaceuticals)	7,775	Sodium bicarbonate 8.4%	2,008
Co-trimoxazole 480mg/5ml	541	T.P.N. Bags	> 290 (Variable with bag contents)

This is not a comprehensive list.

7.2.4 Vasoactive Drugs

Due to their direct vasoconstrictive action on blood vessels, drugs such as adrenaline, noradrenaline, dobutamine, dopamine and vasopressin will reduce the ability of blood vessels in the extravasated area to allow blood to flow freely. This may result in ischaemic injury to the area concerned. If the ischaemia is prolonged or severe, necrosis may develop in the extravasated area.

☞ 7.3 ADMINISTRATION FACTORS AFFECTING EXTRAVASATION

7.3.1   Site Of Administration

The selection of the site is a very important factor when administering an intravenous drug. Areas which have small amounts of subcutaneous tissue are the most likely to be problematic should the drug extravasate. The antecubital fossa and the dorsum of the hand and foot are the most often implicated in extravasation injury and should be avoided when administering irritant or vasoactive drugs and those capable of causing discharge or blistering.

7.3.2   Method Of Venipuncture

This is probably as important as the site of injection. The repeated use of any single vein for venipuncture increases the risk of the drug extravasating to the surrounding tissues. *Venipuncture is a skill, that should not be attempted by anybody who has not completed an approved training course.* Inexperience increases the risk of problems arising from venipuncture.

☛ 7.4 TREATMENT OF EXTRAVASATION

Extravasation should be suspected if:

- ❑ Patient complains of burning, stinging or any discomfort at the injection site.
- ❑ Swelling or leakage is observed at the injection site.
- ❑ Resistance is felt on the plunger of the syringe, if the drug is being given as a bolus.
- ❑ There is an absence of free flow of fluid if an infusion is in progress.

7.4.1 Immediate Action

- ❑ **STOP** the administration of the drug, leaving the cannula in place.
- ❑ Aspirate the residual drug through the cannula.
- ❑ Elevate the limb.
- ❑ Inform the medical staff immediately.

At UCL Hospitals the medical/ surgical team refer cases to the Plastic Surgery team for assessment and advice on treatment at the *earliest opportunity*. The Plastic Surgery team have several techniques available to them to limit the likelihood of extensive tissue damage following extravasation. The sooner these measures are started, the more successful they are likely to be.

7.4.2 Subsequent Action

Careful recording of the following in the medical (and nursing) notes are recommended:

- ❑ Drug(s) involved.
- ❑ Appearance of site.
- ❑ Date and time of the incident.
- ❑ Drug administration technique.
- ❑ Needle size, type and the insertion site.
- ❑ Patient's symptoms and statements.
- ❑ Approximate amount of drug extravasated.
- ❑ Name and signature of nurse/ doctor administering the drug.
- ❑ Doctor notified.
- ❑ Time and date of referral to Plastic Surgery team.
- ❑ Follow-up procedure.

The doctor/ nurse administering the drug should complete an adverse incident form as per Trust policy and any other documentation necessary for patient problems.

It is sometimes necessary to give more than one drug by this method. Not all drugs are suitable for subcutaneous administration because of limited aqueous solubility or extremes of pH. The following simple precautions will minimise the risk of problems of incompatibility and instability.

- Do not mix more then two drugs in a syringe.
- Do not leave anti-emetics running in a syringe pump for more than 24 hours.
- Check with your local pharmacy department for specific stability information before using unusual combinations.

The table below shows the maximum stable concentrations of diamorphine with various agents, made up with water for injection. At concentrations above those shown, there is an increased potential for the mixture to precipitate.

Additive	Maximum stable concentration of additive in syringe pump	Maximum stable concentration of diamorphine in syringe pump	See Note
Cyclizine	10mg/ml	50mg/ml	1
Dexamethasone sodium phosphate	1.6mg/ml	50mg/ml	2
Haloperidol	1.5mg/ml	50mg/ml	
Hyoscine butylbromide	20mg/ml	150mg/ml	
Hyoscine hydrobromide	0.4mg/ml	150mg/ml	
Ketamine (local practice)			3
Methotrimeprazine	10mg/ml	50mg/ml	
Metoclopramide	5mg/ml	150mg/ml	4
Midazolam	5mg/ml	43mg/ml	
Ketorolac	12mg/ml	400mg/ml	5
Octreotide			3

Notes

1 Cyclizine is likely to precipitate in the presence of sodium chloride 0.9%. In addition the solubility of cyclizine is reduced by the concentration of other drugs in solution. Check for precipitation before administration.
  Certain higher concentrations of cyclizine may be compatible with lower concentrations of diamorphine. Contact Pharmacy for details.

2 Check for precipitation before administration.

3 The maximum compatible concentrations of this combination is not known. No formal stability studies have been published.

4 Under some conditions metoclopramide may become discoloured: such solutions should be discarded.

5 Ketorolac and diamorphine should be mixed in sodium chloride 0.9%. The 'maximum' concentrations stated are the maximum concentrations reported in the literature. The absolute maximum compatible concentration of ketorolac and diamorphine is not known.

☞ 9.1 BENEFITS OF INTRAVENOUS ROUTE

The intravenous route has a number of hazards associated with it, and must never be considered lightly.   It should only be used if no other route of administration is appropriate. Situations in which intravenous therapy would be appropriate are when:

❑ The patient is unable to take oral medication, absorb the drug or tolerate the medication

❑ High drug levels are required that cannot be achieved rapidly by another route

❑ Sustained drug levels need to be maintained (such as those achieved by a continuous infusion)

❑ Some drugs cannot be given by another route because of their chemical properties (e.g. are not absorbed from the gut, inactivated by the gut, or are not released from muscle)

❑ An immediate response is required

Drugs administered intravenously avoid having to undergo the process of absorption into the bloodstream compared to other routes e.g. oral drugs are absorbed via the gut mucosa, drugs administered intramuscularly have to be absorbed from the muscle fibres into the bloodstream.

☞ 9.2 IMPACT OF THE FIRST PASS EFFECT

Drugs given orally are usually absorbed in the small intestine and enter the portal system to the liver where they are metabolised. For some drugs metabolism in the liver occurs to such a great extent that little drug reaches the target organ - this is called the first pass effect (or first pass metabolism). Therefore the oral dose for a similar therapeutic effect may need to be higher e.g. verapamil, propranolol, glyceryl trinitrate. For some drugs e.g. lignocaine it is not possible to make an oral formulation because the metabolism is so great.

☞ 9.3 IMPACT OF HALF-LIFE

The half-life ($t_{1/2}$) is the time taken for the concentration of drug in the blood or plasma to fall to half its original value e.g. if a drug has a half-life of 4 hours it means it will take 4 hours for the concentration of the drug in the blood to fall from 10mg/l to 5mg/l. Drugs can have half-lives which are measured in seconds, minutes, hours or days. Therefore drugs with very short half-lives disappear from the bloodstream very quickly and so need to be administered by a continuous infusion to maintain a clinical effect on tissues e.g. dopamine has a half-life of 1-2 minutes and so has to be given as a continuous infusion; when the infusion is stopped the effects it has on the kidney/heart will be lost within minutes. If a drug has a longer half-life it means it can be given as bolus injection instead of an infusion and its effects on the body tissues will last for several hours before another dose is needed.

☞ 9.4 ADVANTAGES AND DISADVANTAGES OF INTRAVENOUS ADMINISTRATION

Advantages

- ❏ Rapid response (e.g. cardiac arrest)
- ❏ Constant therapeutic effect (e.g. continuous infusion)
- ❏ To allow drug administration when the oral route cannot be used (e.g. NBM, patient may aspirate, nausea and vomiting)
- ❏ IM route inappropriate (e.g. small muscle mass, thrombocytopenic, haemophiliacs)
- ❏ To achieve effects unattainable by oral administration (e.g. drug metabolised extensively, non-absorption of drug)
- ❏ To enable drugs to be administered to patients who are unconscious, uncooperative or uncontrollable
- ❏ To allow fluid and electrolyte imbalance to be promptly corrected

Disadvantages

- ❏ Increased risk of toxicity (side effects usually more immediate and severe)
- ❏ Risk of embolism
- ❏ Increased risk of microbial contamination/ infection
- ❏ Risk of extravasation/ phlebitis
- ❏ Risk of particulate contamination
- ❏ Administration hazards (e.g. pain on injection)
- ❏ Risk of fluid overload
- ❏ Problems with compatibility/ stability of drugs/ fluids/ administration sets

☛ 9.5 ROUTES OF INTRAVENOUS ADMINISTRATION

9.5.1 Peripheral Versus Central Vein Administration

Peripheral Vein Administration

Advantages
- ❑ Simpler
- ❑ Cheaper
- ❑ Less traumatic compared to central line
- ❑ Easier to manage for nursing staff

Disadvantages
- ❑ Limited period of use
- ❑ Block more easily
- ❑ Infection
- ❑ Extravasation/ phlebitis
- ❑ One lumen (overcome by 3-way tap but drugs still mix together and tap poses further infection risk)
- ❑ Not suitable for certain drugs

Central Vein Administration

Advantages

- ❑ Administration of hypertonic fluids
- ❑ Administration of other irritant solutions e.g. cytotoxics, TPN, inotropes
- ❑ Rapid administration of large volumes e.g. in shock
- ❑ Long term venous access e.g. cytotoxics, TPN
- ❑ To enable more concentrated solutions of drugs, which would normally need further dilution due to their irritancy, to be given in fluid/ sodium restricted patients e.g. potassium chloride
- ❑ Administration of drugs with a pharmacological action on veins such as vasoconstriction e.g. dopamine, noradrenaline.
- ❑ Can have more than one lumen (e.g. triple lumen) which prevents drugs mixing together

Disadvantages

- ❑ Morbidity associated with central line insertion
- ❑ Takes time and skill to insert
- ❑ Skilled staff required to care for line
- ❑ High infection risk
- ❑ More expensive

Drugs which must be administered centrally include adrenaline, noradrenaline, dopamine and amiodarone.

10. METHODS OF INTRAVENOUS ADMINISTRATION

☞ 10.1 INTRAVENOUS BOLUS

Introduction of a small volume of drug solution into a cannula or the injection site of an administration set. A bolus injection must be administered over 3-5 minutes unless otherwise specified e.g. adenosine which is administered as quickly as possible.

Indications   ❑ To achieve immediate and high drug levels. This may be appropriate when time is limited or in cases of emergency

           ❑ Some drugs are metabolised so quickly, e.g. adenosine, that they must be given as quickly as possible by a bolus otherwise they will exert no clinical effect

Drawbacks   ❑ Tendency to administer the dose too rapidly

           ❑ Damage to the veins, e.g. phlebitis or extravasation, especially with potentially irritant drugs

           ❑ Volume of diluent recommended may not be practical for the time of administration

           ❑ Sudden anaphylactic reaction

           ❑ Increased adverse reactions for some drugs e.g. vancomycin

☞ 10.2 INTERMITTENT INTRAVENOUS INFUSION

Administration of an infusion over a set time period, either as a one-off dose or repeated at specific time intervals. Intermittent infusion of drugs is often a compromise between a bolus injection and continuous infusion. It achieves high plasma concentrations rapidly to ensure clinical efficacy and yet reduces the risks of adverse reactions associated with fast or inappropriate administration of a drug.

☞ 10.3 CONTINUOUS INTRAVENOUS INFUSION

Intravenous administration of a volume of fluid with or without drugs added over 24 hours or over a number of hours to achieve a clinical endpoint. The infusion may be repeated over a period of days. Large volumes (i.e. 250-1,000ml) or small volume infusions (e.g. 50ml of heparin) may be delivered continuously.

Indications	❏ When a constant therapeutic drug concentration is required
	❏ When a drug has a rapid elimination rate or a very short half-life and can only have an effect if given continuously
Drawbacks	❏ Amount of dilution in the infusion fluid required may cause fluid overload in susceptible patients
	❏ Incompatibility problems with the diluent
	❏ Incomplete mixing
	❏ Calculation of rate of administration required using different equipment e.g. solution sets and burettes
	❏ Increased risk of microbial and particulate contamination during the preparation
	❏ Risk of phlebitis and extravasation
	❏ Need for regular monitoring during infusion

11. FORMULATION AND PRESENTATION OF INTRAVENOUS DRUGS

Parenteral drugs differ in the presentations that are available.

☞ 11.1 DRUGS THAT REQUIRE RECONSTITUTION

These include drugs such as amoxycillin which are presented as a dry powder and therefore need to be reconstituted in water for injection or sodium chloride 0.9% before use. Further dilution may be necessary. The advantage of this type of formulation is that it enables prolonged storage of products unstable in solution.

There are a number of disadvantages including:

❏ Reconstitution, which is time consuming, particularly if the preparation is difficult to dissolve
❏ Any manipulations pose the risk of environmental contamination and the risk of microbial contamination of the solution
❏ There is a risk of microbial contamination
❏ Care may be required if the drug is susceptible to 'foaming', as incomplete doses may be withdrawn e.g. teicoplanin
❏ If ampoules require snapping, there is a danger of glass particles getting into the preparation, staff injuries and the risk of drug droplets polluting the environment
❏ Where vials are used there may be pressure difficulties when trying to introduce the diluent or withdraw the reconstituted drug

11.1.2 Equalising Pressure In Vial

Some vials are manufactured with a vacuum inside, and it is important that the effects of this are corrected during reconstitution. If the vial has a vacuum inside it will be obvious when trying to add diluent as the diluent will be 'sucked' into the vial.

If no vacuum is present in the vial, air needs to be removed as the diluent is added. The amount of air drawn back into the syringe should be equal to the volume of diluent added. Before withdrawing the reconstituted drug from the vial, again pressure differences have to be accounted for. Air needs to be added to the vial equal to the amount of drug to be withdrawn.

☛ 11.2 PREPARATIONS IN SOLUTION REQUIRING FURTHER DILUTION BEFORE USE

e.g. ranitidine, amiodarone

The advantages of these preparations are that:

❑ They are already in a liquid form, so reconstitution is unnecessary

The disadvantages include:

❑ Time consuming to draw up and prepare
❑ Prone to vacuum/ pressure problems (if vials)
❑ Can cause glass breakage problems (if ampoules)
❑ Pose the risk of microbial contamination

☛ 11.3 PREPARATIONS AVAILABLE 'READY TO USE' WITHOUT FURTHER DILUTION

These preparations may come in bags or small volume ampoules that can be administered without further dilution, but still require the drug solution to be drawn up into a syringe for administration, e.g. adenosine, gentamicin, metoclopramide. These are convenient to use but still have the disadvantages of:

❑ Hazards associated with microbial contamination
❑ Prone to vacuum/ pressure problems (if vials)
❑ Can cause glass breakage problems (if ampoules)

☛ 11.4 PREPARATIONS 'READY TO USE'

These preparations include infusion bags and pre-filled syringes e.g. sodium chloride 0.9% 500 ml, morphine sulphate 60 mg in 60 ml PCA syringes. They have the advantages of:

❑ No risk of environmental contamination
❑ Minimal microbial contamination
❑ Easy to use
❑ Time saving

12. PROBLEMS ASSOCIATED WITH IV DRUG ADMINISTRATION

☛ 12.1 PAIN ON IV INJECTION

This may be a sign of not following recommended administration advice - check manufacturer's literature, with centres in your local pharmacy drug information department or this guide. It is also important to check the IV site itself for any problems.

Pain on injection can occur with any drugs which are hypertonic [i.e. they have a higher osmotic pressure than plasma (osmolarity > 290mOsmol/l) due to a higher concentration of molecules which causes liquid to pass out of the red blood cells which then shrink], or are administered too quickly or are insufficiently diluted to minimise chemical irritancy. If recommendations are being followed and pain is still a problem, try reducing the rate or increasing the dilution.

Pain can be caused by a wide variety of factors including pH, tonicity and chemical irritancy. The most common examples of drugs that cause pain on injection are listed below:

Erythromycin	Potassium infusions	Sodium bicarbonate 8.4%
Dextrose solutions > 10%	Tetracycline	Phenytoin
Vancomycin		

☞ 12.2 PHLEBITIS AND EXTRAVASATION

12.2.1 Phlebitis

This is a red inflamed vein, corded (hard), with not much flow of drug solution through the vein.

12.2.2 Extravasation (Infiltration, Tissuing)

This is the accidental infiltration of intravenous fluids/ drugs into the subcutaneous tissue (other causes may be physical or chemical). It can occur for a number of reasons and may lead to an inflammatory response and / or pain from the affected tissue which may be immediate or delayed.

It is often thought to be due to cannula being pushed or pulled through the vein and therefore the drug solution leaking out into the tissues. However it can occur from venospasm of the vein caused by administration of an irritant drug causing vasoconstriction and possibly occlusion of the vein. This results in a high back pressure and causes the drug solution to extravasate into the tissue by leaking out of the vein at the point where it was punctured by the cannula.

The most common examples of drugs which can cause more tissue damage if extravasated are given below and are more likely to do so if they are hypertonic (high osmolarity), chemical irritants or have a pH outside 4 - 8 (i.e. strongly acidic or alkaline).

Aciclovir	Calcium chloride	Dopamine	Erythromycin
Sodium Bicarbonate	Phenobarbitone	Vancomycin	Phenytoin
Various cytotoxics			

For further information on the management of extravasation of intravenous drugs refer to Section A 7.

☞ 12.3 FACTORS AFFECTING PATENCY OF IV SITES

12.3.1 Factors Increasing Failure Of IV Sites

- ❑ Infection
- ❑ Irritation - movement
  - cannula material (steel is more irritant than teflon)
  - particles (terminal in-line filters help)
  - irritant drugs (doxorubicin, diazepam, erythromycin, potasssium infusions)
  - pH appears to be an important factor. Extremes of pH i.e. high or low pHs are more likely to be irritant.

28

12.3.2 Factors Decreasing Failure Of IV Sites

❑ Filters
❑ Good practice/ aseptic technique
❑ Neutral solutions
❑ Heparin, topical steroids (blocks inflammatory mechanism), glyceryl trinitrate patches (vasodilation)

☞ 12.4 PROBLEMS WITH RAPID ADMINISTRATION

❑ Usually avoided if administration advice followed.
❑ Wide variety of problems could arise e.g. fluid overload, excessive pharmacological action. Some common problems are listed below.

Drug	Problem
Frusemide	Increased risk of ototoxicity (deafness) at > 4 mg/min
Fusidic acid	Increased risk of haemolysis and hepatotoxicity
Vancomycin	Increased risk of Red Man Syndrome[1] especially if given over less than 1 hour
Sulphonamides	Increased risk of crystalluria (crystals in the urine)
Cimetidine,[2] Ranitidine	Arrhythmias, arrest
Theophylline	Arrhythmias, nausea, vomiting, tachycardia
Potassium chloride	> 20mmol/hour arrhythmias, arrest
Lignocaine	Arrhythmias, arrest
Methylprednisolone sodium succinate	Cardiovascular collapse > 50mg/min
Phenytoin	Arrhythmias, respiratory/cardiac arrest if administered at > 50mg/min

1. Red Man Syndrome - flushing (macular rash), fever, rigors
2. Cimetidine - arrhythmia's appear to be more common compared to ranitidine

☞ 12.5 FACTORS AFFECTING DROP SIZE

The presence of solvents in the drug may affect the drop size of the infusion e.g. amiodarone, etoposide. This can result in inaccuracies if relying on drop counting methods to control the administration rate. Therefore these drugs are best given by devices controlled by volume compared to drop rate (see section 5).

29

☛ 12.6 HIGH SODIUM CONTENT

Sodium may be in the drug as the sodium salt or in the additives as a buffer or may be used as the diluent i.e. sodium chloride 0.9%. Some drugs can have a high sodium content which may need to be taken into consideration when patients are sodium restricted.

Examples:

    ❏ Sodium salts and additives

	Na^+ content
Ceftazidime 2g	4.6mmol/vial
Ciprofloxacin	15.4mmol/100ml

  ❏ Diluent
- IV metronidazole 500mg = 13.6mmol Na^+ per 100ml bag
- Erythromycin depending on volume of sodium chloride 0.9% used as diluent   (e.g. could be 2L/day i.e. 300mmol Na^+)

☛ 12.7 FLUID OVERLOAD

Drugs that require to be diluted in large volumes of diluents for administration may cause problems in patients who are fluid restricted. Fluid overload may also arise where patients are being administered numerous intravenous drugs which may require dilution. Therefore the amount of fluid intake from intravenous drug administration must be considered when prescribing maintenance fluid requirements.

❏ High fluid intake IV may be required for the following drugs:
- Co-trimoxazole (high dose) - Erythromycin
- Sodium fusidate   - Cisplatin
- Cyclophosphamide   - TPN regimens
- Methotrexate (high dose)

☛ 12.8 LAYERING

This phenomenon can occur if there is insufficient mixing of solutions with different densities. The best example of this is the addition of potassium chloride to intravenous infusion bags. If potassium chloride injection is added to glucose 5%, it remains in the bottom of the IV bag as it is denser than glucose. Thus if the two solutions are not mixed thoroughly, there is a high concentration of potassium in the lower part of the IV bag - in this case cardiac arrest could occur as a high concentration of potassium would be delivered in short space of time.

13. FACTORS INFLUENCING DRUG STABILITY AND COMPATIBILITY OF INTRAVENOUS DRUGS

An important aspect of parenteral therapy is to ensure that the patient receives the intended dose of each drug. A proportion of the drug will be lost between the time of preparation of the injection and entry into the bloodstream e.g. if the drug undergoes degradation, precipitates with the diluent, or interacts with the delivery system. It is important to understand the reasons for such losses of potency in order to assess the likely clinical implications.

The following sections will briefly discuss some of these problems.

☞ 13.1 DEGRADATION

13.1.1 In Aqueous Solution

Drugs on reconstitution are relatively unstable in aqueous vehicles and normally degrade by hydrolysis (decomposition of a substance by the chemical action of water). This reaction may be accelerated by a change in pH, due either to the diluent or to a second drug. Such degradation may be minimised and prevented by using the recommended diluent.

For example: erythromycin must be reconstituted with water for injection as it will not dissolve in sodium chloride 0.9% or glucose 5% and then should be diluted in sodium chloride 0.9% and not glucose 5% as it degrades in an acidic pH.

13.1.2 Photodegradation

Photodegradation is the breakdown of a substance by light. It occurs to a significant degree in a small number drugs e.g vitamin A and sodium nitroprusside. Degradation is usually due to ultraviolet light which is found in daylight but not artificial fluorescent light. However sodium nitroprusside is rapidly degraded by both fluorescent and ultraviolet light. Addition to a fat emulsion to TPN almost completely eliminates photodegradation of vitamin A.

Photodegradation of other light sensitive drugs e.g. ciprofloxacin, frusemide, amphoteracin is not clinically important provided direct exposure to strong daylight or sunlight is avoided with the exception of liposomal amphoteracin.

31

☞ 13.2 PRECIPITATION

Precipitated drugs are pharmacologically inactive but are hazardous to the patient. Precipitates can block catheters, damage capillaries and may lead to coronary and pulmonary emboli. The injection of drug precipitates must therefore be avoided.

13.2.1 Causes of Precipitation

pH

The most likely reason for precipitation is the mixing in the infusion container or the infusion line of two injections with very different pHs, especially if one is acid and the other is alkali.

Drug-drug co-precipitation

This occurs most commonly from the mixing of organic anions (ions with a negative charge) and cations (ions with a positive charge) which join together to form ion-pairs. Examples include gentamicin and other aminoglycosides, heparin and some cephalosporins. It is essential to avoid these interactions. Drugs which could form an ion pair should never be allowed to mix in an infusion container, syringe or administration line e.g. flush gentamicin with sodium chloride 0.9% before giving heparin.

Temperature

Most drugs are more soluble as temperature increases. Generally if a refrigerated injection does not precipitate, warming to 37°C (as occurs when an injection passes slowly through the cannula) will not cause precipitation. One exception to this is calcium phosphate, which is less soluble at 37°C than at room temperature. This is important in neonatal TPN, which contains calcium and phosphate, as the two minerals will be heated up to a temperature of > 37°C in the part of the administration line which is in the incubator. If the concentration of the two minerals is too high at this temperature, a precipitate will form.

Mannitol, at concentrations of 15% or greater, crystallise out when exposed to low temperatures. A mannitol solution containing crystals should not be used. If crystallisation occurs, heat the crystals in a water bath at 60-70°C with vigorous shaking periodically and allow the solution to cool to body temperature before use.

☞ 13.3 BINDING OF DRUGS TO PLASTICS

Administration of intravenous drugs relies almost entirely on equipment made from plastics. Some drugs bind to certain plastics. The extent of binding is difficult to predict because it depends on: drug concentration, vehicle, flow rate, available surface area of plastic, type of plastic, temperature, pH and time.

The table shows some clinically relevant examples:

Drug	Plastic affected	Avoided by
Insulin	Any (and glass)	Not adding to infusion, give in syringe pump, at >1unit/ml. Also monitor clinically
Diazepam	PVC	Not using PVC bags and sets. Use polyethylene extension sets and syringe pump (minor losses to syringes - change every 12-24 hours)
Nimodipine	PVC	Using polyethylene extension sets and syringe pump
Nitrates (GTN, ISDN)	PVC, nylon	Not using PVC bags and sets. Use polyethylene extension lines with syringe pumps or polyfusors
Chlormethiazole	PVC, nylon	Not using PVC bags and sets. If PVC sets are used they must be changed at least every 24 hours

☞ 13.4 DESTABILISATION OF PARENTERAL EMULSIONS

Care is necessary to avoid destabilising emulsions in IV lines, junctions and catheters where many injections may mix during administration. Fat emulsions e.g. Intralipid are used widely in parenteral nutrition as an energy source. Other drugs which are prepared as a fat emulsion due to their poor water solubility include propofol and diazepam (Diazemuls).

Fat emulsions can be destabilised by ions with a high positive charge (calcium, magnesium) or by mixing calcium and heparin in the same IV line, for instance in neonatal TPN. Diazemuls may be diluted, but sodium chloride 0.9% rapidly destabilises the emulsion and should not be used.

☞ 13.5 LEACHING OF PLASTICISERS

The presence of oils and surfactants can leach (leak) out toxic plasticisers especially from PVC materials. This can happen if TPN is made in PVC bags. Leaching from administration sets and bags during infusion can also occur. For example cyclosporin: the infusion should be used within 6 hours because the solution contains polyethoxylated castor oil which causes phthalate (a plastic substance) to leach from PVC containers and tubing. If the infusion is administered for more than 6 hours, a low sorbing giving set and a glass bottle should be used to infuse the cyclosporin. Leaching from rubber plungers of plastic syringes may occur and can affect drug stability e.g. asparaginase.

☞ 13.6 BLOOD AND BLOOD PRODUCTS

The Department of Health states the co-administration of blood or concentrated red blood cells with any other drug or vehicle is hazardous. Examples of incompatibility with blood include mannitol solutions (irreversible crenation of red cells), dextrans (rouleaux formation and interference with cross-matching), glucose (clumping of red cells), and oxytocin (inactivated).

In extreme circumstances drugs have been mixed with blood in the catheter. For example, experience seems to show that frusemide can mix safely with blood. In contrast, human serum albumin has been shown to be incompatible with many intravenous infusions. Overall experience remains limited and no studies have been reported.

☞ 13.7 ANAPHYLAXIS

A true allergic reaction resulting in anaphylaxis will occur in a patient who has become sensitised to a drug via an immunological mediated pathway and so must have had previous exposure to the drug. Therefore anaphylaxis will occur on the administration of the second dose rather than on the first dose of the drug. In a patient already sensitised to a specific medication, the risk of an allergic reaction to that medication is greatest when given intravenously and least when given orally. This is thought to be a function of the rate of drug delivery.

Pseudoallergic reactions are drug reactions that exhibit clinical signs and symptoms of an allergic response, but are not immunologically mediated. Unlike true allergic reactions, which require an induction period during which a patient becomes sensitised to an antigen, pseudoallergic reactions can occur on the first exposure to a drug. The development of pseudoallergic reactions may be dose related and become manifested only when large doses of the drug are administered, when the dose is increased, or only when the rate of intravenous administration is increased.

Section B

Drug monographs

(in alphabetical order)

Abbreviations	(See section A 2.4 for further details)
(C) IV infusion	Continuous intravenous infusion
(I) IV infusion	Intermittent intravenous infusion
IV bolus	Intravenous bolus
S/C	Subcutaneous injection
(C) S/C infusion	Continuous subcutaneous infusion
IM	Intramuscular injection
N/S	Sodium chloride 0.9% BP (normal saline)
G	Glucose 5% BP
W	Water for injection (preservative free) BP
G/S	Glucose 4% and sodium chloride 0.18% BP
H	Compound sodium lactate (Hartmann's)
Hep/S	Heparin 10units in 1ml sodium chloride 0.9% – heparinised sodium chloride (e.g. Hepsal)

DRUG AND FORMULATION	METHOD	INSTRUCTION FOR DILUTION AND SUITABLE DILUENT	ADMINISTER OVER	COMMENTS	COMPATIBILITY
Acetazolamide Vial 500mg	IV bolus.	Reconstitute each 500mg with at least 5ml W.	100-500mg/minute.	**Acute Events Which May Accompany Administration** Extravasation may cause tissue damage; for management guidelines see section A 7. **pH:** 9.2 **Flush:** N/S or G.	Do not infuse with other drugs.
	IM. (Not recommended as painful injection).	As above.		**Sodium content:** 2.36mmol/vial. **Displacement:** 0.36ml/500mg. Add 4.64ml of diluent to 500mg vial to give a concentration of 500mg/5ml.	
Acetylcysteine Ampoule 2g/10ml	(C) IV infusion via a volumetric infusion pump.	Dilute with G. Initially give 150mg/kg in 200ml over 15 minutes then 50mg/kg in 500ml over 4 hours followed by 100mg/kg in 1 litre over 16 hours.		**pH:** 7 **Flush:** G or N/S. **Sodium content:** 12.8mmol/10ml. **Other comments** A change in colour of solutions of acetylcysteine to light purple is insignificant.	
Aciclovir (acyclovir) Vial 250mg, 500mg	(I) IV infusion.	Reconstitute 250mg vial with 10ml and 500mg vial with 20ml of W or N/S. Dilute doses up to 500mg in 100ml of N/S or G. For doses greater than 500mg add to 250ml of N/S or G. In fluid restricted patients, reconstitute vial as above and give centrally undiluted via a syringe pump.	Minimum 1 hour.	**Acute Events Which May Accompany Administration** Extravasation may cause tissue damage; for management guidelines see section A 7. **pH:** 11 **Flush:** N/S, G/S or H. **Sodium content:** 1.1mmol/250mg. **Displacement:** negligible. **Other comments** Use infusion within 12 hours.	**Y-site compatible (but see section A 2.6):** ceftazidime, cefuroxime, erythromycin, fluconazole, heparin, imipenem, metronidazole, potassium chloride, tobramycin (both drugs in G), vancomycin. **Incompatible:** dobutamine, dopamine, foscarnet, ondansetron, pethidine.

Notes

a) For abbreviations used in the table see section A 2.4

b) Prepare a fresh infusion every 24 hours unless otherwise specified.

DRUG AND FORMULATION	METHOD	INSTRUCTION FOR DILUTION AND SUITABLE DILUENT	ADMINISTER OVER	COMMENTS	COMPATIBILITY
Adenosine Vial 6mg/2ml	IV bolus.	May be diluted with N/S if necessary.	As quickly as possible.	**Acute Events Which May Accompany Administration** Facial flushing, dyspnoea, tightness in chest. **ECG** monitoring normally required. Resuscitation equipment should be available. **pH:** 6.3-7.3 **Flush:** N/S. **Sodium content:** negligible. **Other comments** If given into an IV line inject as proximally as possible and follow with a rapid N/S flush.	
Addiphos Vial 20ml containing phosphate 40mmol, potassium 30mmol	(I) IV infusion (unlicensed) into a central line via a volumetric infusion pump.	Dilute one vial in 500ml G.	Usual maximum rate 9mmol of phosphate over 12 hours. Faster rates are used in ITU i.e. one vial over 12-24 hours (local practice).	**Acute Events Which May Accompany Administration** Oedema and hypotension, monitor blood pressure. Doses of phosphate exceeding 9mmol/12 hours may cause hypocalcaemia and metastatic calcification. Monitor calcium, phosphate, potassium, other electrolytes and renal function. Pain or phlebitis may occur during peripheral administration of solutions containing more than 30mmol/litre of potassium. **pH:** 6.3-6.4 **Flush:** G. **Sodium content:** 30mmol/vial.	

DRUG AND FORMULATION	METHOD	INSTRUCTION FOR DILUTION AND SUITABLE DILUENT	ADMINISTER OVER	COMMENTS	COMPATIBILITY
Adrenaline Ampoule 1 in 1,000 (1mg/1ml), 1 in 10,000 (1mg/10ml)	(C) IV infusion via syringe or volumetric infusion pump.	Dilute 1mg with 250ml N/S, G, G10%, G/S or H. Unlicensed local practice (ITU) dilute 2mg, 4mg or 8mg to 50ml with N/S or G.	Adjust rate according to response.	**Acute Events Which May Accompany Administration** Arrhythmias. Adrenaline infusions should be used in areas where appropriate cardiovascular monitoring is available (ITU, High Dependency Unit etc). Extravasation may cause tissue damage: for management guidelines see section A 7. **pH:** 2.5-3.6 **Do not flush** replace giving set. **Other comments** The IM route is preferred to S/C as it is more reliable.	**Y-site compatible (but see section A 2.6):** atropine (in G only), chlormethiazole with adrenaline 1:1,000, dobutamine, dopamine, doxapram, frusemide, heparin, insulin, lignocaine, noradrenaline (in G/S or G only), potassium chloride. **Incompatible:** aminophylline.
Min-I-Jet 1 in 10,000 (1mg/10ml),	IV bolus - Emergency use.	Use Min-I-Jet or 1mg/10ml (1 in 10,000) solution.			
1 in 1,000 (1mg/1ml)	IM or S/C. See 'Other comments'.	0.5-1ml of 1 in 1,000 (1mg/1ml).			

Notes

a) For abbreviations used in the table see section A 2.4

b) Prepare a fresh infusion every 24 hours unless otherwise specified.

DRUG AND FORMULATION	METHOD	INSTRUCTION FOR DILUTION AND SUITABLE DILUENT	ADMINISTER OVER	COMMENTS	COMPATIBILITY
Alfentanil Amps 1mg/2ml, 5mg/10ml, 5mg/1ml (for dilution)	IV bolus.	May be diluted with N/S or G.	Minimum 30 seconds in spontaneously breathing patients.	**Acute Events Which May Accompany Administration** Respiratory depression, apnoea and bradycardia. Hypotension may occur if administered too rapidly. Doses above 1mg usually involve significant respiratory depression.	**Y-site compatible (but see section A 2.6):** atracurium, midazolam, mivacurium, pancuronium, propofol. **Incompatible:** alkaline agents, thiopentone.
	(C) IV infusion via syringe pump. Use only in ventilated patients.	Dilute with N/S or G to a convenient volume.	See 'Other comments'	**pH:** 4.3-6 **Flush:** N/S, G. **Other comments** **Anaesthesia:** Adequate plasma levels will only be achieved rapidly if the infusion (0.5-1micrograms/kg/minute) is preceded by a loading dose of 50-100micrograms/kg given as a bolus or fast infusion over 10 minutes. **ITU sedation:** Bolus 15-30micrograms/kg, infusion 20-120micrograms/hour.	
ALG (horse)	See Anti-lymphocyte immunoglobulin horse (ALG Merieux, Lymphoglobuline)				
Allopurinol (unlicensed) Vial 200mg	IV bolus into a fast running drip of N/S or G.	Reconstitute contents of vial with 5ml of W to produce a 40mg/1ml solution. Draw up required dose.	3-5 minutes.	**Acute Events Which May Accompany Administration** Extravasation may cause tissue damage; for management guidelines see section A 7. **pH:** 10.8-11.8 (when reconstituted)	Do not infuse with other drugs.
	(I) IV infusion.	Reconstitute contents of vial with 5ml of W to produce a 40mg/1ml solution. Add dose to at least 50ml of G or N/S	15 minutes.	**Sodium content:** 0.6 mmol/vial. **Flush:** N/S, G.	

DRUG AND FORMULATION	METHOD	INSTRUCTION FOR DILUTION AND SUITABLE DILUENT	ADMINISTER OVER	COMMENTS	COMPATIBILITY
Alphaglobin	See immunoglobulin human normal				
Alprostadil (Prostaglandin E1) Ampoule 500micrograms/1ml	(C) IV infusion via syringe pump.	Dilute with N/S or G usually to between 2 to 20micrograms/1ml.	Variable according to indication. See package insert or specialist protocol for details.	**Acute Events Which May Accompany Administration** Hypotension, monitor arterial pressure; decrease infusion rate immediately if pressure falls significantly. In neonates: apnoea, bradycardia, monitor blood pressure, heart rate, oxygen saturation and respiratory rate. **pH:** Alcoholic solution therefore not applicable. **Do not flush** replace giving set. **Sodium content:** nil.	
Alteplase Vial 20mg, 50mg	Initial IV bolus dose then (I) IV infusion via syringe pump.	Reconstitute 20mg vial with 20ml of W and 50mg vial with 50ml of W.	**MI:** infuse 15mg by initial IV bolus over 1 to 2 minutes, then 0.75mg/kg (maximum 50mg) over 30 minutes and then 0.5mg/kg (maximum 35mg) over 60 minutes.	**Acute Events Which May Accompany Administration** Bleeding at injection site, intracerebral haemorrhage, nausea and vomiting. ECG and haemodynamic monitoring required. **pH:** 7.3 **Sodium content:** nil. **Flush:** N/S. **Other comments** A colourless to pale yellow solution is produced. Foaming may occur, the bubbles will dissipate after standing for a few minutes.	**Y-site compatible (but see section A 2.6):** lignocaine. **Incompatible:** G, dobutamine, dopamine, glyceryl trinitrate, heparin.

Notes

a) For abbreviations used in the table see section A 2.4

b) Prepare a fresh infusion every 24 hours unless otherwise specified.

DRUG AND FORMULATION	METHOD	INSTRUCTION FOR DILUTION AND SUITABLE DILUENT	ADMINISTER OVER	COMMENTS	COMPATIBILITY
Amikacin Vial 100mg/2ml, 500mg/2ml	IV bolus (preferred method).	May be diluted with 10-20ml N/S, G.	2-3 minutes.	**pH:** 4.5 **Flush:** N/S, G. **Sodium content:** 0.14mmol/100mg and 0.72mmol/500mg.	Amikacin may be added to a metronidazole infusion bag. **Y-site compatible (but see section A 2.6):** calcium gluconate, ranitidine.
	(I) IV infusion.	Dilute to 2.5mg/1ml with N/S, G.	30 minutes.		
	IM.	Ready diluted.			**Incompatible:** heparin.
Aminophylline Ampoule 250mg/10ml	(I) IV infusion (initial loading dose) via volumetric infusion pump.	Dilute to 250ml with N/S, G or G/S. Maximum concentration of 25mg/1ml. **Paediatric information:** Dilute to a concentration of 1mg/1ml.	**Adults:** usually 30 minutes (maximum rate 25mg/minute). **Children:** 30 minutes.	**Acute Events Which May Accompany Administration** Tachycardia and hypotension, monitor heart rate and blood pressure. Arrhythmias and convulsions may occur if infusion rate is too fast. Extravasation may cause tissue damage; for management guidelines see section A 7. **pH:** 8.8-10 **Flush:** N/S, G or G/S. **Other comments** Plasma level monitoring is required. **Paediatric information:** Use a syringe or volumetric infusion pump.	**Y-site compatible (but see section A 2.6):** atracurium, dexamethasone, dopamine, erythromycin, flucloxacillin, frusemide, glyceryl trinitrate, heparin, hydrocortisone sodium succinate, lignocaine, metronidazole, pancuronium, phenylephrine, potassium chloride, ranitidine, terbutaline. **Incompatible:** adrenaline, amiodarone, bleomycin, cefotaxime, ciprofloxacin, clindamycin, dobutamine, doxapram, doxorubicin, hydralazine, insulin, morphine, noradrenaline, pethidine.
	(C) IV infusion (maintenance dose) via volumetric infusion pump.	Dilute to 500ml with N/S, G or G/S. Maximum concentration 25mg/1ml. **Paediatric information:** Dilute to a concentration of 1mg/1ml.	**Adults:** typically 0.5mg/kg/hour.		

DRUG AND FORMULATION	METHOD	INSTRUCTION FOR DILUTION AND SUITABLE DILUENT	ADMINISTER OVER	COMMENTS	COMPATIBILITY
Amiodarone Amps 150mg/3ml	IV bolus - Emergency use.	Dilute each 150-300mg with 10-20ml G.	Minimum 3 minutes.	**Acute Events Which May Accompany Administration** IV bolus: patient should be closely monitored e.g. in an intensive care unit, because rapid infusion may	**Y-site compatible (but see section A 2.6):** bretylium, dobutamine, dopamine, glyceryl trinitrate, insulin, isoprenaline,
	(I) IV infusion (loading dose). Administration via a volumetric infusion pump is preferred as amiodarone may reduce drop size. See 'Other comments'.	Dilute loading dose (5mg/kg) in 250ml G.	Over 20 minutes to 2 hours.	cause hypotension and circulatory collapse. Rapid administration may cause hypotension, anaphylactic shock, sweating, nausea and in patients with respiratory failure, bronchospasm and apnoea. Cardiac monitoring required. Thrombophlebitis at the site of infusion. Extravasation may cause tissue damage; for management guidelines see section A 7. **pH:** 3.5-4.5 **Flush:** G. **Sodium content:** nil. **Other comments** Very irritant, when repeated or	lignocaine, metronidazole, noradrenaline, phenylephrine, potassium chloride, procainamide, streptokinase. **Incompatible:** aminophylline, flucloxacillin, frusemide, heparin and N/S.
	(C) IV infusion (maintenance dose) via volumetric infusion pump. See 'Other comments'.	Dilute dose (15mg/kg, maximum 1200mg) in 500ml G.	24 hours.	continuous infusion is anticipated administer via a central line.	

Notes

a) For abbreviations used in the table see section A 2.4

b) Prepare a fresh infusion every 24 hours unless otherwise specified.

DRUG AND FORMULATION	METHOD	INSTRUCTION FOR DILUTION AND SUITABLE DILUENT	ADMINISTER OVER	COMMENTS	COMPATIBILITY
Amoxycillin Vial 250mg, 500mg	IV bolus (preferred method).	Reconstitute 250mg with 5ml W and 500mg with 10ml W.	3-4 minutes.	**pH:** 8.6-8.8 **Flush:** N/S. <u>Sodium content:</u> 3.2mmol/1g. <u>Displacement:</u> 0.2ml/250mg (0.4ml/500mg). Add 4.8ml diluent to 250mg vial to give a concentration of 50mg in 1ml or 9.8ml diluent to 250mg vial to give a concentration of 25mg in 1ml.	<u>Y-site compatible (but see section A 2.6):</u> metronidazole. <u>Incompatible:</u> aminoglycosides.
	(I) IV infusion.	Reconstitute as above then dilute with 50-100ml N/S.	30-60 minutes.		
	IM.	Reconstitute 250mg with 1.5ml of W and 500mg with 2.5ml of W. Substitute lignocaine 1% for W if pain is a problem.		**Other comments** Use infusion within 8 hours. A transient pink colouration or slight opalescence may appear during reconstitution. Reconstituted solutions may be a pale straw colour.	

DRUG AND FORMULATION	METHOD	INSTRUCTION FOR DILUTION AND SUITABLE DILUENT	ADMINISTER OVER	COMMENTS	COMPATIBILITY
Amphotericin Vial 50mg (50,000 units)	(I) IV infusion via a volumetric infusion pump.	Reconstitute vial with 10ml W to give a 5mg/1ml solution. Add phosphate buffer, see 'Other comments'. Dilute volume required with 50 times as much G to produce a maximum concentration of 10mg/100ml for peripheral administration. For central administration: dilutions up to 40mg/100ml have been used (unlicensed).	2-4 hours. Rarely up to 6 hours. The CSM advise administration of a test dose on initiation of therapy. Typically administer 1mg over 20-30 minutes and observe the patient for a further 30 minutes.	<u>**Acute Events Which May Accompany Administration**</u> Rapid infusion may increase side effects. Peripheral administration may cause local venous pain at the injection site with phlebitis and thrombophlebitis. This may be relieved by the addition of heparin 500-1,000units to the amphotericin bag. Fever (sometimes with shaking chills) may be relieved by adding pethidine 50mg to the amphotericin bag. Other side effects include headache and vomiting. **pH:** 5.7 **Flush:** with G before and after administration. **Sodium content:** negligible. **Displacement:** negligible. **Other comments** The manufacturers recommend that the pH of G must exceed 4.2 to prevent precipitation. To ensure this, add phosphate buffer to G before amphotericin is added. The phosphate buffer label should state the volume of phosphate to be added to the amphotericin. To reduce nephrotoxicity, prehydrate with N/S 1 litre.	May be mixed in an infusion bag with pethidine (local practice) or heparin. <u>**Y-site compatible (but see section A 2.6):**</u> heparin, magnesium sulphate, sodium bicarbonate. <u>**Incompatible:**</u> N/S, benzylpenicillin, calcium salts, cimetidine, dobutamine, dopamine, fluconazole, foscarnet, frusemide, gentamicin, methyldopate, ondansetron, potassium chloride, ranitidine.

Notes

a) For abbreviations used in the table see section A 2.4
b) Prepare a fresh infusion every 24 hours unless otherwise specified.

44

DRUG AND FORMULATION	METHOD	INSTRUCTION FOR DILUTION AND SUITABLE DILUENT	ADMINISTER OVER	COMMENTS	COMPATIBILITY
Amphotericin lipid complex (Abelcet) Vial 100mg/20ml	(I) IV Infusion via a volumetric infusion pump.	Withdraw the required dose into a syringe and add to 500ml of G through the 5 micron filter needle provided. In fluid restricted or paediatric patients add to 250ml of G.	2.5mg/kg/hour For test dose see 'Other comments'.	**Acute Events Which May Accompany Administration** Apnoea. **pH:** 5-7 (undiluted) **Flush:** before and after administration with G. **Sodium content:** 3.13mmol/vial. **Other comments** It is advisable to administer a test dose on initiation of therapy even if the patient had previously tolerated an alternative amphotericin formulation. Typically 1ml (5mg) in 100ml of G should be infused IV over 15 minutes.	**Incompatible** N/S. Do not mix with other drugs or fluids.
Amphotericin liposomal (AmBisome) Vial 50mg	(I) IV infusion.	Add 12ml W to 50mg vial and shake vigorously for at least 15 seconds. Resulting amphotericin concentration 4mg/1ml. Dilute dose required through the 5 micron filter provided with between 1 and 19 parts of G by volume, to give a final concentration of between 0.2mg/1ml and 2mg/1ml.	30-60 minutes. For test dose see 'Other comments'.	**pH:** 5-6 **Flush:** before and after administration with G. **Sodium content:** less than 0.5mmol/vial. **Other comments** It is advisable to administer a test dose on initiation of therapy even if the patient had previously tolerated an alternative amphotericin formulation. A small dose (e.g. 1-5mg) should be infused over about 10 minutes and the patient carefully observed for 30 minutes. Protect infusion from light.	**Incompatible** N/S. Do not mix with other drugs or fluids.

DRUG AND FORMULATION	METHOD	INSTRUCTION FOR DILUTION AND SUITABLE DILUENT	ADMINISTER OVER	COMMENTS	COMPATIBILITY
Anti-lymphocyte immunoglobulin horse (ALG Merieux, Lymphoglobuline) (unlicensed) Vial 100mg/5ml	(I) IV infusion via a volumetric infusion pump into a large vein.	Dilute each vial of 100mg with at least 50ml of N/S. The usual volume is 250ml-500ml in total.	8 hours (local practice). For test dose see 'Other comments'.	**Acute Events Which May Accompany Administration** Local painful inflammation, erythema, pruritis, fevers, chills. Anaphylaxis may occur (reduced arterial pressure, respiratory distress, fever and urticaria). Symptoms decrease as the course progresses. Regular observations and **ECG** monitoring are required for the first 3 days. If well tolerated, 4 hourly observations for subsequent infusions are required. **pH:** 7 (undiluted)	Do not infuse with other drugs including G.
	Deep IM (likely to be very painful).			**Flush:** N/S. **Other comments** The manufacturers recommend that a test dose is given and that a corticosteroid and an anti-histamine be given IV one hour before infusion is started. Local practice on the UCLH Renal Unit is not prescribe a test dose but to prescribe PRN paracetamol, chlorpheniramine and to have hydrocortisone and adrenaline available.	

Notes

a) For abbreviations used in the table see section A 2.4

b) Prepare a fresh infusion every 24 hours unless otherwise specified.

DRUG AND FORMULATION	METHOD	INSTRUCTION FOR DILUTION AND SUITABLE DILUENT	ADMINISTER OVER	COMMENTS	COMPATIBILITY
Anti-thymocyte immunoglobulin rabbit (ATG Merieux, Thymoglobuline) (unlicensed) Vial 25mg	(I) IV infusion via a volumetric infusion pump into a large vein.	Reconstitute with W (diluent provided) to 5mg/1ml. Dilute each vial with a minimum of 50ml N/S or G (N/S used in practice). The usual volume is 250ml-500ml in total.	6-8 hours (local practice). For test dose see 'Other comments'.	**Acute Events Which May Accompany Administration** Fever, shivering, arthralgia, skin rashes and less frequently anaphylactic reactions (hypotension, respiratory distress, urticaria). Regular observations and ECG monitoring are required for the first 3 days. If well tolerated, 4 hourly observations for subsequent infusions are required. **Other comments** The manufacturers recommend that a test dose is given and that a corticosteroid and an anti-histamine be given IV one hour before infusion is started. Local practice on the UCLH Renal Unit is not prescribe a test dose but to prescribe PRN paracetamol, chlorpheniramine and to have hydrocortisone and adrenaline available. **pH:** 5.5-5.9 **Flush:** N/S.	Do not infuse with other drugs.

47

DRUG AND FORMULATION	METHOD	INSTRUCTION FOR DILUTION AND SUITABLE DILUENT	ADMINISTER OVER	COMMENTS	COMPATIBILITY
Anti-thymocyte immunoglobulin rabbit (ATG Fresenius) (unlicensed) Vial 40mg/2ml, 100mg/5ml	(I) IV infusion via a volumetric infusion pump into a large vein.	Dilute each daily dose with 250ml-500ml N/S.	6-8 hours (local practice). For test dose see 'Other comments'.	**Acute Events Which May Accompany Administration** Fever, shivering, arthralgia, skin rashes and less frequently anaphylactic reactions (hypotension, respiratory distress, urticaria). Half hourly observations and ECG monitoring are required for the first 3 days. If well tolerated, 4 hourly observations for subsequent infusions are required. Extravasation may cause tissue damage; for management guidelines see section A 7. **pH:** 3.7 **Flush:** N/S. **Other comments** The manufacturers recommend that a test dose is given and that a corticosteroid and an anti-histamine be given IV one hour before infusion is started. Local practice on the UCLH Renal Unit is not prescribe a test dose but to prescribe PRN paracetamol, chlorpheniramine and to have hydrocortisone and adrenaline available.	Do not infuse with other drugs including G.

Notes

a) For abbreviations used in the table see section A 2.4

b) Prepare a fresh infusion every 24 hours unless otherwise specified.

48

DRUG AND FORMULATION	METHOD	INSTRUCTION FOR DILUTION AND SUITABLE DILUENT	ADMINISTER OVER	COMMENTS	COMPATIBILITY
Aprotinin Vial 500,000 kallikrein inactivator units (K.I.U)/50ml	IV bolus (initial loading dose).	Provided ready diluted. May be diluted with N/S, G or G/S.	Maximum rate 10ml of original solution /minute. For test dose see 'Other comments'.	<u>**Acute Events Which May Accompany Administration**</u> Hypersensitivity reactions. Peripheral administration may occasionally cause thrombophlebitis. **pH:** 5-7 **Flush:** N/S. **Sodium content:** 7.7mmol/50ml.	Do not infuse with other drugs.
	(C) IV infusion.	As above.	20-50ml of original solution /hour. For test dose see 'Other comments'.	<u>**Other comments**</u> Patient should be supine for administration. The manufacturers recommend that an initial 5ml of loading dose should be infused slowly to test for allergic reactions.	
Argipressin (synthetic vasopressin) Amp 20units/1ml	(I) and (C) IV peripheral infusion.	Usual dilution: add 20units to 100ml G. In fluid restriction dilute with G to a maximum concentration of 20units/20ml (unlicensed).	**For GI haemorrhage:** Loading dose 20units over a minimum of 15 minutes. Maintenance dose 0.4units per minute.	<u>**Acute Events Which May Accompany Administration**</u> Anaphylactic shock may occur. Monitor blood pressure, respiration and heart rate. Argipressin may precipitate angina and there is a risk of myocardial infarction. Extravasation may cause tissue damage; for management guidelines see section A 7. **pH:** 2.5-5.4	
	IM or S/C.	Ready diluted.		**Flush:** N/S or G. **Other comments** Use a glyceryl trinitrate 10mg patch with IV argipressin administration to reduce risk of	

DRUG AND FORMULATION	METHOD	INSTRUCTION FOR DILUTION AND SUITABLE DILUENT	ADMINISTER OVER	COMMENTS	COMPATIBILITY
				coronary spasm.	
Atenolol Vial 5mg/10ml	IV bolus.	May be diluted with N/S, G or G/S.	Maximum rate 1mg/minute.	**Acute Events Which May Accompany Administration** Severe bradycardia and hypotension, monitor heart rate and blood pressure.	
	(I) IV infusion via volumetric infusion pump.	Dilute with N/S, G or G/S.	20 minutes.	Can cause conduction defects, monitor **ECG.** If infused too quickly there is a higher incidence of the above effects. **pH:** 6 **Flush:** N/S, G or G/S. **Sodium content:** approximately 1.3-1.8mmol/5mg.	
ATG (rabbit)	See anti-thymocyte immunoglobulin (Merieux) and (Fresenius)				
Atracurium Ampoule 25mg/2.5ml, 50mg/5ml, 250mg/25ml	IV bolus.	May be administered undiluted or may be diluted with G, G/S or N/S.	1 minute.	**Acute Events Which May Accompany Administration** Histamine release may produce flushing and rarely bronchospasm. **pH:** 3.5 **Flush:** N/S.	**Y-site compatible (but see section A 2.6):** alfentanil, aminophylline, co-trimoxazole (both drugs in G), dopamine, fentanyl, gentamicin, glyceryl trinitrate, heparin, isoprenaline, midazolam, morphine, potassium chloride, sodium nitroprusside. **Incompatible:** alkaline agents, propofol, thiopentone.
	(C) IV infusion via syringe pump.	May be administered undiluted or can be diluted with G, G/S or N/S.	300-600 micrograms/kg/hour.		

Notes

a) For abbreviations used in the table see section A 2.4

b) Prepare a fresh infusion every 24 hours unless otherwise specified.

50

DRUG AND FORMULATION	METHOD	INSTRUCTION FOR DILUTION AND SUITABLE DILUENT	ADMINISTER OVER	COMMENTS	COMPATIBILITY
Atropine Ampoule 600micrograms/1ml Min-I-Jet 1mg/10ml Pre-filled syringe 3mg/10ml	IV bolus, IM or S/C.	Ready diluted.	Give rapidly since slow IV administration may cause paradoxical slowing of the heart.	**Acute Events Which May Accompany Administration** Arrhythmias and paradoxical slowing of the heart, monitor **ECG** if feasible. Extravasation may cause tissue damage; for management guidelines section A 7. **pH:** 3-6.5 **Flush:** N/S.	**Y-site compatible (but see section A 2.6):** adrenaline (in G only), buprenorphine, dobutamine, frusemide, heparin, midazolam, morphine, propofol, potassium chloride. **Incompatible:** alkaline agents.
Augmentin	See co-amoxiclav				

DRUG AND FORMULATION	METHOD	INSTRUCTION FOR DILUTION AND SUITABLE DILUENT	ADMINISTER OVER	COMMENTS	COMPATIBILITY
Azathioprine Vial 50mg	(1) IV infusion (preferred method) via volumetric infusion or syringe pump.	**Handle as for cytotoxic drugs.** Reconstitute with a minimum of 5-15ml W and then dilute with 20-200ml N/S or G/S.	30-60 minutes.	**Acute Events Which May Accompany Administration** Extravasation may cause tissue damage; for management guidelines see section A 7. **pH:** 10-12 (pH 8-9.5 when diluted with N/S or G/S). **Flush:** N/S or G. **Sodium content:** 0.2mmol/vial. **Displacement:** negligible. **Other comments** Discard if any turbidity or crystallisation occurs.	Do not infuse with other drugs.
	IV bolus into a Y-site of a fast flowing N/S or G drip. Flush with at least 50ml N/S or G/S as very irritant.	**Handle as for cytotoxic drugs.** Reconstitute with a minimum of 5-15ml W.	Usually 3-5 minutes. Minimum 1 minute.		

Notes

a) For abbreviations used in the table see section A 2.4

b) Prepare a fresh infusion every 24 hours unless otherwise specified.

52

DRUG AND FORMULATION	METHOD	INSTRUCTION FOR DILUTION AND SUITABLE DILUENT	ADMINISTER OVER	COMMENTS	COMPATIBILITY
Azithromycin (unlicensed) Vial 500mg	(I) IV infusion.	Reconstitute with 4.8ml W to produce a 100mg/1ml solution. Remove the required volume of the solution and further dilute in 100-500ml N/S to a concentration not greater than 2mg/1ml.	30-60 minutes.	**Flush:** N/S.	Do not infuse with other drugs.
Azlocillin Vial 1g, 2g, 5g	IV bolus for doses of 1g or 2g.	Reconstitute 1g with 10ml of W and 2g with 20ml of W.	3-5 minutes.	**Acute Events Which May Accompany Administration** Local irritation at injection site. **pH:** 6-8 (reconstituted). **Flush:** N/S. **Sodium content:** 1g contains 2.17mmol, 2g contains 4.33mmol, 5g contains 10.84mmol.	**Y-site compatible (but see section A 2.6):** N/S, G, G/S, heparin. **Incompatible:** aminoglycosides, metronidazole.
	(I) IV infusion for doses of 5g.	Reconstitute 5g with 50ml of W.	20-30 minutes.	**Other comments** Discard unused solution after 6 hours.	

DRUG AND FORMULATION	METHOD	INSTRUCTION FOR DILUTION AND SUITABLE DILUENT	ADMINISTER OVER	COMMENTS	COMPATIBILITY
Benzylpenicillin Vial 600mg (1 megaunit)	IV bolus (preferred method).	Reconstitute each 600mg with 4-10ml W, N/S or G.	**Adults:** 3-5 minutes. Maximum rate 300mg/minute.	**Acute Events Which May Accompany Administration** Rapid administration may cause CNS irritation leading to convulsions. Anaphylaxis. **pH:** 6.8 **Flush:** N/S or G. **Sodium content:** 1.68mmol/vial. **Displacement:** 0.4ml/600mg.	**Y-site compatible (but see section A 2.6):** heparin. **Incompatible:** amphotericin, flucloxacillin, gentamicin, tranexamic acid.
	(I) IV infusion.	Reconstitute as above then dilute each 600mg with a minimum of 10ml N/S or G (suggested volume 100ml).	30-60 minutes.	Add 3.6ml of diluent to 600mg vial to give a concentration of 600mg/4ml.	
	IM	Reconstitute each 600mg with 1.6ml W.			
Bretylium Ampoule 500mg/10ml	IV bolus - Emergency use only.	Ready diluted.	1 minute.	**Acute Events Which May Accompany Administration** Hypotension and tachycardia, monitor blood pressure and ECG. **pH:** 6 **Flush:** N/S or G. **Sodium content:** nil.	**Y-site compatible (but see section A 2.6):** amiodarone, digoxin, dobutamine, dopamine, esmolol, lignocaine.
	(I) IV infusion via syringe pump.	Dilute 1 part bretylium with a minimum of 4 parts N/S or G by volume i.e. less than or equal to 10mg/1ml.	Minimum 8 minutes; preferably 15-30 minutes.		
	(C) IV infusion via syringe pump.	As above.	1-2mg/minute.	**Other comments**	

Notes

a) For abbreviations used in the table see section A 2.4

b) Prepare a fresh infusion every 24 hours unless otherwise specified.

54

DRUG AND FORMULATION	METHOD	INSTRUCTION FOR DILUTION AND SUITABLE DILUENT	ADMINISTER OVER	COMMENTS	COMPATIBILITY
	IM. See 'Other comments'.	Ready diluted.		The IM route can cause necrosis, vary site of injection and limit volume to 5ml on any one site.	
Bumetanide Ampoule 1mg/2ml, 2mg/4ml, 5mg/10ml	IV bolus (for doses up to 2mg).	May be diluted with N/S or G if necessary. May be given undiluted.	Maximum rate 1mg/minute.	**Acute Events Which May Accompany Administration** Hypotension, monitor blood pressure.	**Y-site compatible (but see section A 2.6):** doxapram, frusemide, morphine, pethidine. **Incompatible:** dobutamine.
	(I) IV infusion (for doses above 2mg).	Dilute to a suitable volume with G, N/S or G/S to a maximum concentration of 1mg in 10ml.	30 minutes.	Myalgia is common if doses above 2mg are given as a bolus. **pH:** 6.8-7.8 **Flush:** N/S.	
	IM.	Ready diluted.		**Sodium content:** negligible. **Other comments** Discard if cloudiness develops.	
Buprenorphine Ampoule 300microgram/1ml	IV bolus.	May be diluted with N/S or G	At least 2 minutes.	**Acute Events Which May Accompany Administration** Hypotension and respiratory depression, monitor blood pressure and respiration rate.	**Y-site compatible (but see section A 2.6):** atropine, droperidol. **Incompatible:** diazepam, lorazepam.
	(C) IV infusion (unlicensed).	As above.	25-250 micrograms/hour.	Sedation, monitor sedation scores. Extravasation may cause tissue damage; for management guidelines see section A 7. **pH:** 3.5-5.5 **Flush:** N/S.	
	Deep IM injection.	Ready diluted.		**Sodium content:** nil.	

DRUG AND FORMULATION	METHOD	INSTRUCTION FOR DILUTION AND SUITABLE DILUENT	ADMINISTER OVER	COMMENTS	COMPATIBILITY
Calcium chloride Min-I-Jet 10% 10ml containing 6.8mmol calcium/10ml.	IV bolus - Emergency use.	Ready diluted.	**Adults:** Maximum rate 1-2ml/minute.	**Acute Events Which May Accompany Administration** Rapid IV administration may cause vasodilation, decreased blood pressure, bradycardia, cardiac arrhythmias, syncope and cardiac arrest. Very irritant; always administer slowly. Extravasation may cause tissue damage; for management guidelines see section A 7. **pH:** 5.5-7.5 **Flush:** N/S.	**Compatibility/Incompatibility:** see calcium gluconate.
Calcium folinate	See folinic acid				
Calcium gluconate Ampoule 10%, 10ml containing 2.2mmol calcium/10ml.	IV bolus - Emergency use.	Ready diluted.	**Adults:** Maximum rate 0.44mmol calcium (2ml of 10%)/minute. **Neonates:** Maximum rate 0.022mmol calcium (0.1ml of 10%)/ minute.	**Acute Events Which May Accompany Administration** Rapid IV administration may cause vasodilation, decreased blood pressure, bradycardia, cardiac arrhythmias, syncope and cardiac arrest. Extravasation may cause tissue damage; for management guidelines see section A 7. **pH:** 5-7 **Flush:** N/S.	**Y-site compatible (but see section A 2.6):** amikacin, dobutamine, heparin, lignocaine, magnesium sulphate, noradrenaline, potassium chloride. **Incompatible:** amphotericin, bicarbonates, clindamycin, fluconazole, hydrocortisone sodium succinate, pamidronate, phosphates, tartrates.
	(I) IV or (C) IV infusion.	Dilute with N/S, G or G/S.			
	IM.	Maximum volume 5ml.			

Notes

a) For abbreviations used in the table see section A 2.4

b) Prepare a fresh infusion every 24 hours unless otherwise specified.

DRUG AND FORMULATION	METHOD	INSTRUCTION FOR DILUTION AND SUITABLE DILUENT	ADMINISTER OVER	COMMENTS	COMPATIBILITY
Campath-1G (unlicensed) See vial label for total amount of protein and volume of solution.	(I) IV infusion via a syringe pump through a 5 micron in-line filter (local practice).	Dilute required dose with either 50ml or 500ml N/S.	Give first dose over 8 hours. Subsequent doses over 2-4 hours.	**Acute Events Which May Accompany Administration** May provoke hypersensitivity reactions, particularly with first dose, including fever chills, rigors, nausea and urticaria. These might be controlled by reducing the rate of infusion. More severe reactions have occurred e.g. bronchospasm and hypotension. **Flush:** N/S. **Other comments** Campath-1G should be stored frozen (below -30°C). When thawed, the antibody solution should be clear and free from particles or precipitate, though it may be slightly opalescent. Once thawed, it should not be re-frozen, but may be kept for up to 48 hours at 2-8°C. The infusion must be given with care, particularly the first dose. Premedication with paracetamol is recommended and on occasion IV hydrocortisone and chlorpheniramine.	Do not infuse with other drugs.

DRUG AND FORMULATION	METHOD	INSTRUCTION FOR DILUTION AND SUITABLE DILUENT	ADMINISTER OVER	COMMENTS	COMPATIBILITY
Cefotaxime Vial 500mg, 1g, 2g	IV bolus (preferred method).	Reconstitute 500mg with 2ml, 1g with 4ml and 2g with 10ml W.	3-5 minutes.	**pH:** 5-7 **Flush:** N/S or G. **Sodium content:** 2.09mmol/1g.	Cefotaxime may be added to a metronidazole infusion bag. **Y-site compatible (but see section A 2.6):** heparin. **Incompatible:** alkaline agents, aminoglycosides, aminophylline.
	(I) IV infusion.	Reconstitute as above then dilute each 1 or 2g with 40-100ml N/S, G or G/S.	20-60 minutes.	**Displacement:** 0.2ml/500mg vial. Add 1.8ml of diluent to 500mg vial to give a concentration of 500mg in 2ml (250mg in 1ml). **Other comments** Reconstituted cefotaxime forms a straw coloured solution. Variations in the intensity of colour do not indicate changes in potency or safety.	
	IM.	Reconstitute 500mg with 2ml, 1g with 4ml and 2g with 10ml W. Doses of 2g should be divided and administered at different sites.			
Ceftazidime Vial 250mg, 500mg, 1g, 2g	IV bolus (preferred method). Maximum dose 2g.	Reconstitute 250mg with a minimum of 2.5ml, 500mg with 5ml, 1g and 2g with 10ml W, N/S or G.	3-5 minutes.	**pH:** 5-8 **Flush:** N/S, G or G/S. **Sodium content:** 2.3mmol/1g. **Displacement:** 0.25ml/250mg. Add 2.25ml of diluent to 250mg vial to give a concentration of 250mg/2.5ml (100mg in 1ml).	Ceftazidime may be added to a metronidazole infusion bag. **Y-site compatible (but see section A 2.6):** aciclovir, heparin, hydrocortisone sodium succinate, potassium chloride. **Incompatible:** aminoglycosides, fluconazole, sodium bicarbonate,
	(I) IV infusion.	Reconstitute as above then dilute to 50-100ml with N/S or G.	Maximum 30 minutes.		
	Deep IM.	Reconstitute 250mg with 1ml W, 500mg with 1.5ml W and 1g with 3ml W. 2g not recommended.			

58

Notes

a) For abbreviations used in the table see section A 2.4

b) Prepare a fresh infusion every 24 hours unless otherwise specified.

DRUG AND FORMULATION	METHOD	INSTRUCTION FOR DILUTION AND SUITABLE DILUENT	ADMINISTER OVER	COMMENTS	COMPATIBILITY
Cefuroxime Vial 250mg, 750mg, 1.5g	IV bolus (preferred method).	Reconstitute 250mg with at least 2ml W, 750mg with 6ml W and 1.5g with 15ml W. May be diluted with N/S, G or G/S.	3-5 minutes.	<u>**pH:**</u> 6-8.5 <u>**Flush:**</u> N/S, G or G/S. <u>**Sodium content:**</u> 1.8mmol/750mg. <u>**Displacement:**</u> 0.18ml/250mg vial. Add 2.32ml of diluent to 250mg vial to give a concentration of 250mg/2.5ml (100mg in 1ml).	Cefuroxime may be added to a metronidazole infusion bag. <u>**Y-site compatible (but see section A 2.6):**</u> aciclovir, foscarnet, heparin, morphine.
	(I) IV infusion.	Reconstitute as above then dilute to 50 - 100ml with N/S or G.	Maximum 30 minutes.		<u>**Incompatible:**</u> aminoglycosides, doxapram, fluconazole, sodium bicarbonate. .
	IM.	Reconstitute 250mg with 1ml W, 750mg with 3ml W (1.5g for IV administration only).			
Chloramphenicol sodium succinate Vial 1g	IV bolus.	Reconstitute vial with 9.2ml of W, N/S or G (100mg/1ml). Other dilutions may be used see package insert for details. Suggested maximum concentration 100mg/1ml.	1 minute.	<u>**Acute Events Which May Accompany Administration**</u> Vomiting, respiratory difficulties, pale cyanotic skin and hypotension. <u>**pH:**</u> 5.5-7 <u>**Flush:**</u> N/S. <u>**Sodium content:**</u> 3.14mmol/1g.	<u>**Y-site compatible (but see section A 2.6):**</u> dopamine, heparin, hydrocortisone sodium succinate. <u>**Incompatible:**</u> phenothiazines e.g. prochlorperazine, tetracyclines.
	(I) IV infusion.	Reconstitute as above then dilute with N/S, G or G/S.	Minimum time 10 minutes.	<u>**Displacement:**</u> 0.8ml/1g vial. Add 9.2ml diluent to 1g vial to give a concentration of 1g/10ml (100mg in 1ml).	
	IM. See 'Other comments'.	Reconstitute vial with 1.7ml of W, N/S or G (400mg/1ml). Other dilutions may be used see package insert for details.		<u>**Other comments**</u> Absorption from the IM route may be slow and unpredictable.	
Chlormethiazole	(C) IV infusion	Ready diluted.	Status	<u>**Acute Events Which May Accompany**</u>	<u>**Y-site compatible (but see**</u>

DRUG AND FORMULATION	METHOD	INSTRUCTION FOR DILUTION AND SUITABLE DILUENT	ADMINISTER OVER	COMMENTS	COMPATIBILITY
Intravenous infusion bottle 0.8% 500ml containing chlormethiazole edisylate 8mg/1ml	via volumetric infusion or syringe pump. See 'Other comments' for further information.		**epilepticus:** **Adults:** initially 5-15ml/minute. **Children:** Initially 0.01ml/kg/ minute. **Acute alcohol withdrawal:** Initially 3-7.5ml/min, reduce to 0.5-1ml/min or lower. For further information and other indications see package insert.	**Administration** Rapid administration may cause apnoea, hypotension and tachycardia. Prolonged infusion increases the risk of accumulation leading to deep unconsciousness and respiratory arrest. Resuscitation equipment and intubation facilities must be readily available. Thrombophlebitis may occur at the injection site which is not responsive to steroids/heparin. Monitor blood pressure, heart rate, respiration rate, sedation score. **Other comments** **Adults:** Polyethylene giving sets and Teflon cannula are preferred although PVC sets may be used if necessary for administration with volumetric infusion pumps. Change giving set/extension set and syringes every 24 hours. **Children:** Polyethylene syringes and extension sets and Teflon cannulae are recommended. If administration via volumetric pump is necessary see above under adults. Change giving set/extension set and syringes every 24 hours. **pH:** 6-7.5 **Flush:** N/S. **Sodium content:** 16mmol/500ml.	**section A 2.6):** adrenaline 1:1,000, co-trimoxazole, dopamine, doxapram, frusemide, magnesium sulphate, mannitol, metronidazole, naloxone, pancuronium, phenytoin, potassium chloride, suxamethonium, sodium bicarbonate 8.4%. Electrolytes Na, K, Ca and Cl can be added to infusion if necessary as infusion only contains Na$^+$ 16mmol/500ml and no other electrolytes.

Notes

a) For abbreviations used in the table see section A 2.4

b) Prepare a fresh infusion every 24 hours unless otherwise specified.

60

DRUG AND FORMULATION	METHOD	INSTRUCTION FOR DILUTION AND SUITABLE DILUENT	ADMINISTER OVER	COMMENTS	COMPATIBILITY
Chloroquine Sulphate Ampoule 272.5mg/5ml ≡ 200mg/5ml chloroquine base	(C) IV infusion (preferred method).	Dilute with N/S.		**Acute Events Which May Accompany Administration** Rapid IV infusion may result in cardiovascular toxicity and other symptoms of acute overdose e.g. hypotension and arrhythmias.	Do not infuse with other drugs.
	IM (should be avoided in paediatric patients).	Ready diluted.		**pH:** 5.5-6.6 **Flush:** N/S.	
	S/C.	Ready diluted.			
Chlorphenira-mine Ampoule 10mg/1ml	IV bolus.	Dilute with 5-10ml N/S, W, (or patient's own blood).	Minimum 1 minute.	**Acute Events Which May Accompany Administration** Rapid injection may cause transitory hypotension or CNS stimulation.	Do not administer with other drugs.
	IM or S/C.	Ready diluted.		**pH:** 4-5.2 **Flush:** N/S.	
Chlorpromazine	(I) IV infusion	Dilute 25-50mg with 500ml-	1mg/minute.	**Acute Events Which May Accompany**	Do not infuse with other drugs.

61

DRUG AND FORMULATION	METHOD	INSTRUCTION FOR DILUTION AND SUITABLE DILUENT	ADMINISTER OVER	COMMENTS	COMPATIBILITY
Ampoule 25mg/1ml, 50mg/2ml	via volumetric infusion pump (unlicensed).	1 litre N/S.		**Administration** Hypotension especially with rapid administration. Keep patient supine and monitor blood pressure. **pH:** 5-6.5 (undiluted) **Flush:** N/S. **Sodium content:** negligible. **Other comments** Very irritant; avoid peripheral administration if possible.	
	IV bolus (unlicensed).	Dilute to 1mg/1ml with N/S.	**Adults:** Maximum rate 1mg/minute **Children:** Maximum rate 500micrograms /minute.		
	IM.	Ready diluted.	Slowly by deep injection in to the upper outer quadrant of the buttock.		
	IV bolus via central line (unlicensed local practice - ITU).	Ready diluted.	Slowly, monitor blood pressure.		

Notes

a) For abbreviations used in the table see section A 2.4

b) Prepare a fresh infusion every 24 hours unless otherwise specified.

DRUG AND FORMULATION	METHOD	INSTRUCTION FOR DILUTION AND SUITABLE DILUENT	ADMINISTER OVER	COMMENTS	COMPATIBILITY
Cholecystokinin (CCK) (unlicensed) Vial 75 ivy dog units (I.D.U.)	IV bolus.	Dissolve contents of vial in 7.5ml N/S to give a concentration of 10 I.D.U./1ml. Avoid vigorous shaking. Use immediately.	Over 1-5 minutes depending on indication. For test dose see 'Other comments'.	**Acute Events Which May Accompany Administration** Rapid administration may cause sensations of warmth and flushing. Risk of allergic reactions as porcine derived. Transient nausea, abdominal cramps usually subside within 10 minutes. Extravasation may cause tissue damage; for management guidelines see section A 7. **pH:** 3-6 **Flush:** N/S. **Other comments** Give an intravenous test dose of 1 I.D.U., wait 1 minute. If there is no allergic response administer the recommended dose.	Do not administer with other drugs.
Cimetidine Ampoule 200mg/2ml	(I) IV infusion (preferred method). See 'Other comments'.	Dilute with N/S or G usually to 100ml.	30-60 minutes.	**Acute Events Which May Accompany Administration** Cardiac arrhythmias, monitor blood pressure and heart rate. Rapid IV administration may cause arrhythmias.	**Y-site compatible (but see section A 2.6):** TPN.
	IV bolus See 'Other comments'.	Dilute with 20ml N/S.	Minimum 2 minutes; preferably 5 minutes or longer.	**pH:** 5.6-6.4 (in infusion bag), 4.5-6 (ampoule). **Flush:** N/S or G. **Other comments** (I) IV infusion must be used for doses over 200mg or if there is cardiovascular impairment.	
	(C) IV infusion.	Dilute with N/S or G to a convenient volume.	50-100mg/ hour.		
	IM.	Ready diluted.	100-200mg		
Ciprofloxacin	(I) IV infusion.	Ready diluted.		**pH:** 3.9-4.5	**Y-site compatible (but see**

DRUG AND FORMULATION	METHOD	INSTRUCTION FOR DILUTION AND SUITABLE DILUENT	ADMINISTER OVER	COMMENTS	COMPATIBILITY
Vial 100mg/50ml, Infusion bag 200mg/100ml, 400mg/200ml			over 30-60 minutes. 400mg over 60 minutes.	**Flush:** N/S. **Sodium content:** 15.4mmol/100ml.	**section A 2.6):** G, N/S, G/S, cyclosporin, dobutamine, dopamine, digoxin, gentamicin, lignocaine, metronidazole, potassium chloride, tobramycin. **Incompatible:** aminophylline, flucloxacillin, frusemide, heparin, hydrocortisone sodium succinate, methylprednisolone, phenytoin.
Clarithromycin Vial 500mg	(I) IV infusion in large proximal vein.	Reconstitute each vial with 10ml W, producing a solution containing 50mg/1ml. Dilute resultant solution with N/S or G to produce a final solution of approximately 2mg/1ml (e.g. 500mg in 250ml).	60 minutes.	**Acute Events Which May Accompany Administration** Phlebitis, tenderness and inflammation at injection site. Rapid infusion may cause arrhythmias. **pH:** 5 (in N/S) **Flush:** N/S or G. **Sodium content:** negligible.	Do not infuse with other drugs.

Notes

a) For abbreviations used in the table see section A 2.4

b) Prepare a fresh infusion every 24 hours unless otherwise specified.

DRUG AND FORMULATION	METHOD	INSTRUCTION FOR DILUTION AND SUITABLE DILUENT	ADMINISTER OVER	COMMENTS	COMPATIBILITY
Clindamycin Ampoule 300mg/2ml, 600mg/4ml	(I) IV infusion (maximum dose 1.2g).	Dilute to a concentration of 6mg/1ml with G or N/S (300mg in 50ml of G or N/S). Maximum concentration is 12mg/1ml.	Maximum rate: 30mg/minute (1.2g over at least 45 minutes).	**Acute Events Which May Accompany Administration** Thrombophlebitis, erythema, pain and swelling. **pH:** 5.5-7 **Flush:** N/S.	**Y-site compatible (but see section A 2.6):** foscarnet, potassium chloride, zidovudine (both drugs in G). **Incompatible:** aminophylline, calcium salts, magnesium sulphate, phenytoin, thiopentone.
	(C) IV infusion doses above 1.2g.	Seek advice.			
	IM (maximum 600mg).	Ready diluted.			
Clonazepam Ampoule 1mg/1ml	IV bolus - Emergency use into large vein of the antecubital fossa.	Immediately before use dilute each 1mg in 1ml with 1ml W, to produce a 1mg in 2ml solution.	Maximum rate 30 seconds / 1mg.	**Acute Events Which May Accompany Administration** Hypotension, apnoea, monitor blood pressure and respiratory function. Salivary or bronchial hypersecretion. Extravasation may cause tissue damage; for management guidelines see section A 7. **pH:** 3.5-4.5	
	(I) or (C) IV infusion via volumetric infusion pump.	Dilute up to 3mg in 250ml of G, G/S or N/S.		**Flush:** N/S. **Sodium content:** nil. **Other comments** Discard unused infusion after 12 hours.	
Clonidine	IV bolus.	May be diluted with N/S or G.	Give slowly preferably over	**Acute Events Which May Accompany Administration**	

DRUG AND FORMULATION	METHOD	INSTRUCTION FOR DILUTION AND SUITABLE DILUENT	ADMINISTER OVER	COMMENTS	COMPATIBILITY
Ampoule 150micrograms/1ml			3-5 minutes.	Bradycardia, monitor heart rate and blood pressure. Rapid administration may produce transient hypertension and then hypotension. **pH:** 4-4.5 **Flush:** N/S. **Sodium content:** negligible.	
Colistin Vial 1MU	(I) IV infusion.	Reconstitute with 10ml W or N/S then dilute further with N/S or G. Usual final volume 50-100ml. Maximum volume 500ml.	Usually over 30-60 minutes. Maximum 6 hours.	**Flush:** N/S. **Sodium content:** 0.23mmol/1 million units. **Displacement:** negligible. **Other comments** Use infusion within 6 hours.	Do not infuse with other drugs.
Co-amoxiclav Vial 600mg,	IV bolus (preferred method).	Reconstitute 600mg with 10ml and 1.2g with 20ml W.	3-4 minutes.	**pH:** 8.8-9 **Flush:** N/S. **Sodium content:** 1.6mmol/600mg, 3.1mmol/1.2g.	**Incompatible:** aminoglycosides.
containing amoxycillin 500mg and clavulanic acid 100mg and 1.2g containing amoxycillin 1g and clavulanic acid 200mg	(I) IV infusion.	Reconstitute as above then dilute 600mg to 50ml and 1.2g with 100ml N/S.	30-40 minutes.	**Potassium content:** 0.5mmol/600mg, 1mmol/1.2g. **Displacement:** 0.5ml/600mg, 0.9ml/1.2g. Add 9.5ml W to 600mg vial to give a concentration of 600mg/10ml. Add 19.1ml W to 1.2g vial to give a concentration of 1.2g/20ml. **Other comments** Discard unused infusion after 4 hours.	

Notes

a) For abbreviations used in the table see section A 2.4

b) Prepare a fresh infusion every 24 hours unless otherwise specified.

DRUG AND FORMULATION	METHOD	INSTRUCTION FOR DILUTION AND SUITABLE DILUENT	ADMINISTER OVER	COMMENTS	COMPATIBILITY
Co-trimoxazole Ampoule 480mg/5ml, 960mg/10ml containing trimethoprim 1 part to sulphamethoxazole 5 parts	(I) IV infusion.	Dilute each 480mg (5ml) to 125ml, 960mg (10ml) to 250ml, 1440mg (15ml) to 500ml, 1920mg (20ml) and 2400mg (25ml) to 500-1000ml with N/S, G, or G/S.	Give over at least 60-90 minutes. Give over 2 hours if causing nausea.	**Acute Events Which May Accompany Administration** Nausea and vomiting. Thrombophlebitis at site of infusion. Localised pain and irritation during infusion. Extravasation may cause tissue damage; for management guidelines see section A 7. **pH:** 9-10.5 **Flush:** N/S. **Sodium content:** 1.64mmol/480mg. **Other comments** More stable in G than N/S. Discard diluted infusion within 6 hours of preparation. Monitor all infusions carefully for cloudiness and precipitate formation.	**Y-site compatible (but see section A 2.6):** aciclovir (both drugs in glucose), atracurium (both drugs in glucose), chlormethiazole, magnesium sulphate (both drugs in glucose), morphine (both drugs in glucose), pancuronium (both drugs in glucose). **Incompatible:** insulin.
	(I) IV infusion via a syringe pump into a central line (unlicensed).	Local practice on UCLH HIV and Haematology wards: Doses less than 40ml (3840mg) in 500ml G. Doses of 40ml (3840mg) or more in 1000ml N/S. Undiluted (local practice).	90 minutes to 2 hours. 90 minutes. Give over 2 hours if causing nausea.		
Cyclizine	IV bolus.	May be diluted with W.	3-5 minutes.	**Acute Events Which May Accompany**	**Compatibility in syringe pump:**

DRUG AND FORMULATION	METHOD	INSTRUCTION FOR DILUTION AND SUITABLE DILUENT	ADMINISTER OVER	COMMENTS	COMPATIBILITY
Ampoule 50mg/1ml				**Administration** Hypotension and tachycardia, monitor blood pressure and heart rate. Pain at injection site. Extravasation may cause tissue damage; for management guidelines see section A 7. **pH:** 3.3-3.7	with diamorphine see section A 8 for details. Morphine 1mg/1ml and cyclizine <2mg/1ml in N/S. **Incompatible:** All solutions of pH greater than 6.8. Octreotide.
	(I) or (C) IV or S/C infusion (unlicensed).	May be diluted with W or N/S (local practice).		**Flush:** W or N/S. **Sodium content:** nil. **Other comments**	
	IM.	Ready diluted.		W is more stable than N/S.	

Notes

a) For abbreviations used in the table see section A 2.4
b) Prepare a fresh infusion every 24 hours unless otherwise specified.

DRUG AND FORMULATION	METHOD	INSTRUCTION FOR DILUTION AND SUITABLE DILUENT	ADMINISTER OVER	COMMENTS	COMPATIBILITY
Cyclosporin Ampoule 50mg/1ml, 250mg/5ml	(I) IV infusion via syringe or volumetric infusion pump.	Dilute 1 in 20 up to 1 in 100 by volume with N/S or G i.e. 1ml (50mg) in 20-100ml.	2-6 hours Administration rates may vary in accordance with trial protocols or local practice see 'Other comments'.	<u>**Acute Events Which May Accompany**</u> <u>**Administration**</u> Anaphylactic reactions, continuously observe patient for first 30 minutes following initiation of infusion and subsequently monitor patient frequently. **pH:** 6-7 **Flush:** N/S. **Other comments:** Use infusion within 6 hours because the solution contains polyethoxylated castor oil which causes phthalate leaching from PVC containers and tubing. If infusion is administered for more than 6 hours, use an IVAC Low Sorbing Tubing code 59953 and infuse cyclosporin in a 500ml G glass bottle. Protect ampoules from light. Prepared infusions do not need to be protected from light. Plasma level monitoring is required.	<u>**Y-site compatible (but see**</u> <u>**section A 2.6):**</u> ciprofloxacin.
Dalteparin Pre-filled syringe 2,500iu/0.2ml, 5,000iu/0.2ml	S/C.	Ready diluted.		**pH:** 5-7.5 **Flush:** N/S or G. **Other comments** IV administration is only licensed for the prevention of clotting in the extracorporeal circulation during haemodialysis or haemofiltration in patients with chronic renal insufficiency or acute renal failure.	
Ampoule 10,000iu/4ml,	IV bolus.	May be diluted with N/S or G.	Dependent on indication.	The S/C route is licensed for unstable angina, surgical thromboprophylaxis and treatment of DVT.	
10,000iu/1ml	(I) or (C) IV infusion.	May be diluted with N/S or G.	Dependent on indication.		

DRUG AND FORMULATION	METHOD	INSTRUCTION FOR DILUTION AND SUITABLE DILUENT	ADMINISTER OVER	COMMENTS	COMPATIBILITY
Dantrolene Vial 20mg	IV bolus.	Reconstitute 20mg with 60ml W.	Give rapidly.	**Acute Events Which May Accompany Administration** Give centrally if possible because of high pH. If given peripherally care is needed to avoid extravasation as it may cause tissue damage; for management guidelines see section A 7.	**Incompatible:** do not give with other drugs or infusion fluids including G and N/S.
	(I) IV infusion (used for prophylaxis of pre-operative malignant hyperthermia).	As above, do not dilute further.	1 hour.	**pH:** 9.5 **Flush:** W. **Sodium content:** 2mmol/20mg vial. **Other comments** Discard 6 hours after reconstitution.	

Notes

a) For abbreviations used in the table see section A 2.4

b) Prepare a fresh infusion every 24 hours unless otherwise specified.

DRUG AND FORMULATION	METHOD	INSTRUCTION FOR DILUTION AND SUITABLE DILUENT	ADMINISTER OVER	COMMENTS	COMPATIBILITY
Desferrioxamine Vial 500mg	(I) or (C) IV infusion.	Reconstitute each 500mg with 5ml W to give a 10% solution. This may be further diluted with N/S, G or G/S.	**Chronic iron overload:** 8-12 hours. Some patients may require administration over 24 hours. **Maintenance haemo-dialysis / filtration:** Infuse IV dose in 100ml N/S over the last 30-60 minutes of dialysis.	**Acute Events Which May Accompany Administration** Anaphylactoid reactions, fever and muscle aches. IV bolus may lead to circulatory collapse. Concentrations of greater than 10% will increase the risk of local skin reactions if administered S/C. **pH:** 3.5-6.5 **Flush:** N/S. **Displacement:** 0.4ml/500mg. Add 4.6ml diluent to 500mg vial to give a concentration of 500mg in 5ml. **Other comments** Discard infusion if cloudy.	Hydrocortisone sodium succinate may be added to the infusion bag (local practice). **Incompatible:** heparin.
	(I) or (C) S/C infusion.	As above.			
	IM.	Reconstitute each 500mg with 5ml W. Can inject dose in two injections.			

DRUG AND FORMULATION	METHOD	INSTRUCTION FOR DILUTION AND SUITABLE DILUENT	ADMINISTER OVER	COMMENTS	COMPATIBILITY
Desmopressin Ampoule 4micrograms/1ml	IV bolus.	Ready diluted.	5 minutes.	**Acute Events Which May Accompany Administration** Tachycardia and hypotension, monitor blood pressure continuously during infusions. Fluid overload likely, restrict fluid intake and check body weight regularly.	
	(I) IV infusion.	Dilute dose with 50ml N/S. In children less than 10kg dilute dose with 10ml of N/S.	20-30 minutes.	**pH:** 4 **Flush:** N/S. **Other comments** Doses of less than 4micrograms (1ml) should not be diluted but measured with a suitably graduated syringe. Dilution may result in loss of desmopressin by absorption onto glass or plastic.	
	IM or S/C.	Ready diluted.			
Dexamethasone (as sodium phosphate) Vial 8mg/2ml, 500micrograms/1ml (unlicensed)	IV bolus.	May be diluted with N/S or G.	Minimum 3 minutes.	**Acute Events Which May Accompany Administration** Rapid administration may cause perianal itching. Serious anaphylactoid reactions e.g. bronchospasm have occurred. **pH:** 7-8.5 **Flush:** N/S. **Sodium content:** 0.021mmol/1ml. **Other comments** The last dose should preferably be given before 6pm to avoid insomnia.	**Y-site compatible (but see section A 2.6):** aminophylline, diamorphine, fluconazole, heparin, granisetron, metoclopramide, metronidazole, morphine. **Compatibility in syringe pump:** with diamorphine see section A 8 for details. **Incompatible:** octreotide, phenothiazines e.g. prochlorperazine, vancomycin.
	(I) IV infusion.	Dilute in 100ml N/S or G.	15 minutes.		

Notes

a) For abbreviations used in the table see section A 2.4

b) Prepare a fresh infusion every 24 hours unless otherwise specified.

DRUG AND FORMULATION	METHOD	INSTRUCTION FOR DILUTION AND SUITABLE DILUENT	ADMINISTER OVER	COMMENTS	COMPATIBILITY
Diamorphine Ampoule 5mg, 10mg, 30mg, 100mg, 500mg	S/C or IM.	Dilution not required.			**Compatibility in syringe pump:** see section A 8 for details. **Incompatible:** alkaline agents.
	IV bolus.	Reconstitute 5mg, 10mg, 30mg and 100mg ampoules with 1ml W. Reconstitute 500mg ampoule with 2ml W. May be diluted with G or N/S (preferably G).	3-5 minutes (local practice).	**Acute Events Which May Accompany Administration** Severe respiratory depression, apnoea, hypotension, peripheral circulatory collapse, chest wall rigidity, cardiac arrest and anaphylactic shock. Monitor blood pressure, heart and respiratory rate. **Flush:** N/S or G. **Sodium content:** nil. **Displacement:** negligible. **Other comments** Infusion is more stable in G than N/S.	
	(C) IV infusion via syringe pump.	As above for reconstitution. Dilute with G or N/S (preferably G) to a convenient volume.			
	(C) S/C infusion via syringe pump.	To reconstitute ampoule see IV bolus. Dilute with W if to be added to other compatible drugs. Dilute with N/S if not to be mixed with other drugs. Dilute to a convenient volume.			
	IM or S/C.	As for IV.			

DRUG AND FORMULATION	METHOD	INSTRUCTION FOR DILUTION AND SUITABLE DILUENT	ADMINISTER OVER	COMMENTS	COMPATIBILITY
Diazepam emulsion Ampoule 10mg/2ml	IV bolus.	Ready diluted.	5mg/minute.	**Acute Events Which May Accompany Administration** Aponoea and hypotension, monitor respiratory rate and blood pressure. Circulatory and respiratory depression, monitor heart and respiratory rate. **pH:** 8 **Flush:** N/S.	<u>Y-site compatible (but see section A 2.6):</u> N/S.
	(C) IV Infusion via a syringe pump.	Dilute with G or G 10% to achieve a concentration within the range 0.1-0.4mg/1ml (i.e. 1-4ml in 50ml G).	Titrate rate to response. Maximum rate 125micrograms /kg/hour.	<u>Other comments</u> Discard solution after 6 hours. Diazepam emulsion causes less local pain and thrombophlebitis compared to diazepam injection. Adsorption may occur to PVC infusion equipment. This occurs to a greater extent with diazepam injection.	

Notes
a) For abbreviations used in the table see section A 2.4
b) Prepare a fresh infusion every 24 hours unless otherwise specified.

DRUG AND FORMULATION	METHOD	INSTRUCTION FOR DILUTION AND SUITABLE DILUENT	ADMINISTER OVER	COMMENTS	COMPATIBILITY
Diazepam Ampoule 10mg/2ml	(C) IV Infusion - not recommended use diazepam emulsion.			**Acute Events Which May Accompany Administration** Aponoea and hypotension, monitor respiratory rate and blood pressure. Circulatory and respiratory depression, monitor heart and respiratory rate.	**Y-site compatible (but see section A 2.6):** dobutamine. **Incompatible:** buprenorphine, doxapram, frusemide, flucloxacillin, glycopyrronium, heparin, ranitidine.
	IV bolus - not recommended use diazepam emulsion.			There is a higher incidence of vein irritation compared with diazepam emulsion. Extravasation may cause tissue damage; for management guidelines see section A 7. **pH:** 6.2-6.9	
	IM. Only use when oral or IV dosing is not possible or advisable because absorption is variable.	Ready diluted.		**Other comments** Discard unused solution within 6 hours. Avoid contact with polyvinyl chloride administration sets. **Sodium content:** nil	

DRUG AND FORMULATION	METHOD	INSTRUCTION FOR DILUTION AND SUITABLE DILUENT	ADMINISTER OVER	COMMENTS	COMPATIBILITY
Diazoxide Ampoule 300mg/20ml	IV bolus - Emergency use only (maximum dose 150mg).	Do not dilute.	Give rapidly (less than 30 seconds).	**Acute Events Which May Accompany Administration** Hyperglycaemia, monitor blood glucose levels regularly. Reflex tachycardia in the first few minutes after injection. Pain or a feeling of warmth along injected vein. Extravasation may cause tissue damage; for management guidelines see section A 7. **pH:** 11.6 **Flush:** N/S. **Sodium content:** 15mmol/300mg. **Other comments** Dose may be repeated after 5-15 minutes if necessary. Slow administration reduces the antihypertensive response.	

Notes

a) For abbreviations used in the table see section A 2.4

b) Prepare a fresh infusion every 24 hours unless otherwise specified.

DRUG AND FORMULATION	METHOD	INSTRUCTION FOR DILUTION AND SUITABLE DILUENT	ADMINISTER OVER	COMMENTS	COMPATIBILITY
Diclofenac Ampoule 75mg/3ml	(I) IV infusion.	Buffer 100-500ml of N/S or G with sodium bicarbonate solution (0.5ml 8.4% or 1ml 4.2%). Add one ampoule of diclofenac to the infusion bag.	25-50mg over 15-60 minutes. 75mg over 30-120 minutes.	**Acute Events Which May Accompany Administration** IM injection may cause site reactions, abscesses and local necrosis. **pH:** 7.8-9 **Flush:** N/S or G. **Sodium content:** negligible.	Do not infuse with other drugs.
	(C) IV infusion.	As above.	Approximately 5mg/hour.	**Other comments** Maximum duration of parenteral treatment is 2 consecutive days. Administer IM injection by deep intragluteal injection into the upper quadrant. If necessary use alternate buttock for second injection.	
	IM. See 'Other comments'.	Ready diluted.			
Dicobalt edetate Ampoule 300mg/20ml	IV bolus.	Ready diluted.	Maximum rate 300mg/minute. If patient's condition is less serious give dose over 5 minutes.	**Acute Events Which May Accompany Administration** Can cause hypotension and tachycardia. **pH:** 4-7.5 **Sodium content:** nil. **Other comments** Each dose may be followed immediately with 50ml G 50%.	<u>Y-site compatible (but see section A 2.6):</u> G, W.

DRUG AND FORMULATION	METHOD	INSTRUCTION FOR DILUTION AND SUITABLE DILUENT	ADMINISTER OVER	COMMENTS	COMPATIBILITY
Digibind Vial 38mg	(I) IV infusion.	Reconstitute vial with 4ml of W. May be diluted with N/S to a suitable volume. Administer through 0.2 micron sterile disposable filter.	30 minutes.	**Acute Events Which May Accompany Administration** Continuous ECG monitoring for 24 hours after administration of Digibind. Significant hypokalaemia can occur, monitor potassium levels. Allergic reactions, rash, shaking and chills without fever can occur. **pH:** 6-8 **Flush:** N/S.	Do not infuse with other drugs.
	IV bolus (use if cardiac arrest seems imminent).	Reconstitute vial with 4ml of W.	3-5 minutes.	**Sodium content:** 0.47mmol/vial. **Other comments** The reconstituted vial should be stored in the refrigerator and used within 4 hours.	
Digoxin Ampoule 500microgram/2ml, 100micrograms/1ml (paediatric)	(I) IV infusion via syringe or volumetric infusion pump (preferred method).	Dilute 1 part digoxin with at least 4 parts N/S, G or G/S. Volume of final solution for adults is usually 50-100ml (maximum 500ml).	Usually 2 or more hours. Minimum time: 10-20 minutes.	**Acute Events Which May Accompany Administration** Arrhythmias, monitor heart rate and **ECG** recommended. Rapid injection may cause vasoconstriction and transient hypertension, monitor blood pressure. **pH:** 6.7-7.3	**Y-site compatible (but see section A 2.6):** bretylium, ciprofloxacin, flecainide, flucloxacillin, frusemide, heparin, insulin, lignocaine, morphine, potassium chloride, streptokinase, verapamil.
	IV bolus.	Dilute 1 part digoxin with at least 4 parts N/S, G or G/S.	Minimum time: 5-10 minutes	**Flush:** N/S. **Other comments**	**Incompatible:** dobutamine, doxapram, foscarnet.
	IM. See 'Other comments'.	Ready diluted.		The IM route is rarely justified as it causes severe local irritation and results in unreliable absorption.	

Notes

a) For abbreviations used in the table see section A 2.4

b) Prepare a fresh infusion every 24 hours unless otherwise specified.

DRUG AND FORMULATION	METHOD	INSTRUCTION FOR DILUTION AND SUITABLE DILUENT	ADMINISTER OVER	COMMENTS	COMPATIBILITY
Disopyramide Ampoule 50mg/5ml	IV bolus (maximum dose 150mg).	Ready diluted.	Minimum time: 5 minutes. Maximum rate 30mg/minute	**Acute Events Which May Accompany Administration** If given too quickly profuse sweating and cardiovascular depression may occur. Monitor blood pressure and **ECG.** Preferred route is peripheral as central administration may potentially increase risk of hypotension and cardiac arrest.	Do not infuse with other drugs.
	(C) IV infusion following loading dose as IV bolus. Use syringe or volumetric infusion pump.	Dilute with N/S or G.	20-30mg/hour or 0.4mg/kg/hour.	**pH:** 4-5 **Flush:** N/S. **Other comments** Maximum dose 300mg in first hour and 800mg in 24 hours (including loading dose).	

DRUG AND FORMULATION	METHOD	INSTRUCTION FOR DILUTION AND SUITABLE DILUENT	ADMINISTER OVER	COMMENTS	COMPATIBILITY
Dobutamine Ampoule 250mg/20ml	(C) IV infusion via syringe pump.	Dilute to 5mg/1ml with N/S or G. Concentrations of up to 10mg/1ml have been used via a central line (unlicensed local practice).		<u>**Acute Events Which May Accompany**</u> <u>**Administration**</u> Heart rate, rhythm and arterial blood pressure should be closely monitored. The use of dobutamine should be restricted to areas where full haemodynamic monitoring is available. Extravasation may cause tissue damage; for management guidelines see section A 7. **pH:** 3.5-4 **Do not flush** replace giving set. **Sodium content:** negligible. <u>**Other comments**</u> Solution may turn pink. This is due to a slight oxidation of the drug and is harmless.	<u>**Y-site compatible (but see**</u> <u>**section A 2.6):**</u> adrenaline, amiodarone, atropine, bretylium, calcium chloride, calcium gluconate, ciprofloxacin, diazepam, dopamine, glyceryl trinitrate, hydralazine, isoprenaline, lignocaine, magnesium sulphate, noradrenaline (local practice), pancuronium, phenylephrine, potassium chloride, procainamide, sodium nitroprusside (both drugs in N/S). **Incompatible:** aciclovir, alteplase, aminophylline, amphotericin, bumetanide, digoxin, frusemide, sodium bicarbonate and other strong alkaline agents.

80

Notes

a) For abbreviations used in the table see section A 2.4

b) Prepare a fresh infusion every 24 hours unless otherwise specified.

DRUG AND FORMULATION	METHOD	INSTRUCTION FOR DILUTION AND SUITABLE DILUENT	ADMINISTER OVER	COMMENTS	COMPATIBILITY
Dopamine Ampoule 200mg/5ml Infusion 400mg/250ml	(C) IV infusion via a volumetric infusion or syringe pump. See 'Other comments'.	Dilute with N/S, G, G10% or G/S to a suggested maximum concentration of 1.6mg/1ml (800mg in 500ml). Concentrations up to 8mg/1ml have been used (unlicensed). A dilution of 200mg in 50ml is used routinely on the ICUs (local practice). See 'Other comments' for choice of route of administration.		**Acute Events Which May Accompany Administration** When administered peripherally, extravasation can produce local vasoconstriction leading to severe tissue hypoxia and ischaemia; for general treatment guidelines see section A 7. If extravasation occurs irrigate affected area with 5-10mg phentolamine in 10-15ml N/S. Observe infusion site carefully. ECG monitoring is usually required but is not essential for low dose (1-3micrograms/kg/min) infusions. **pH:** 2.5-4.5 **Do not flush** - replace giving set. **Sodium content:** 0.52mmol/200mg. **Other comments** Administration via a central line is advisable and for concentrations > 2mg/1ml is essential. If given peripherally use a dilute solution (1.6mg/1ml or less) and administer via a large vein. **Paediatric information:** Use a central venous line for concentrations > 2mg/1ml and doses over 10micrograms/kg/minute.	**Y-site compatible (but see section A 2.6):** adrenaline, aminophylline, amiodarone, atracurium, bretylium, chloramphenicol, chlormethiazole, ciprofloxacin, dobutamine, doxapram, glyceryl trinitrate, heparin, insulin, labetalol, lignocaine, mannitol, noradrenaline, potassium chloride, sodium nitroprusside. **Incompatible:** aciclovir, alteplase, amphotericin, sodium bicarbonate, other alkaline agents.

DRUG AND FORMULATION	METHOD	INSTRUCTION FOR DILUTION AND SUITABLE DILUENT	ADMINISTER OVER	COMMENTS	COMPATIBILITY
Doxapram Ampoule 100mg/5ml, Infusion bottle 1g in 500ml of glucose 5%	(C) IV infusion via volumetric infusion pump.	Provided ready diluted 1g in 500ml G.	Rate control recommended. **Adults:** Usual maximum rate 4mg/minute.	**Acute Events Which May Accompany Administration** Moderate increase in blood pressure and slight increase in heart rate. Extravasation may cause tissue damage; for management guidelines see section A 7. **pH:** 3-5	**Y-site compatible (but see section A 2.6):** adrenaline, bumetanide, chlormethiazole, dopamine, potassium chloride, terbutaline. **Incompatible:** alkaline agents e.g. aminophylline, cefuroxime, diazepam, digoxin, frusemide, ketamine, sodium bicarbonate.
	IV bolus.	May be diluted with N/S, G or G10%.	Minimum 30 seconds.	**Flush:** N/S or G. **Other comments** Single bolus injections should not exceed 1mg/kg.	
Droperidol Ampoule 10mg/2ml	IV bolus.	May be diluted with N/S or G.	3-5 minutes.	**Acute Events Which May Accompany Administration** Rapid administration may cause hypotension and tachycardia. Monitor blood pressure and heart rate. Extravasation may cause tissue damage; for management guidelines see section A 7.	**Y-site compatible (but see section A 2.6):** buprenorphine, fentanyl, glycopyrronium, metoclopramide, midazolam, mivacurium, morphine. **Incompatible:** barbiturates, frusemide, heparin, thiopentone.
	(C) IV infusion via volumetric infusion or syringe pump.		1-3mg/hour.	**pH:** 2.7-4.7 **Flush:** N/S or G. **Sodium content:** nil.	
	IM.	Ready diluted.			

Notes

a) For abbreviations used in the table see section A 2.4

b) Prepare a fresh infusion every 24 hours unless otherwise specified.

DRUG AND FORMULATION	METHOD	INSTRUCTION FOR DILUTION AND SUITABLE DILUENT	ADMINISTER OVER	COMMENTS	COMPATIBILITY
EloHaes (formally Elohes) (Hetastarch 6% in N/S) Infusion bag 500ml	(I) or (C) IV infusion. For rapid administration a blood administration set can be used.	Ready diluted.	Dependent upon patient requirements.	**Acute Events Which May Accompany Administration** Extravasation may cause tissue damage; for management guidelines see section A 7. **pH:** 3.5 **Flush:** N/S or G. **Sodium content:** 154mmol/L.	**Incompatible:** gentamicin.
Ephedrine Ampoule 30mg/1ml	IV bolus.	Dilute to 3mg in 1ml with N/S, G or G/S.	3-5 minutes.	**Acute Events Which May Accompany Administration** Hypertension, monitor blood pressure. CNS disturbances. **pH:** 4.5-7 **Flush:** N/S	**Incompatible:** hydrocortisone sodium succinate, phenobarbitone, thiopentone.
	IM.	Ready diluted.			

DRUG AND FORMULATION	METHOD	INSTRUCTION FOR DILUTION AND SUITABLE DILUENT	ADMINISTER OVER	COMMENTS	COMPATIBILITY
Epoprostenol (prostacyclin) Vial 500,000nanograms	(C) IV infusion via syringe or volumetric infusion pump.	Reconstitute using the 50ml diluent provided to prepare a concentrate containing 10,000nanograms/1ml. Prime the filter with concentrate before measuring the required dose. Dilute each 1 part concentrate, using filter provided, with a maximum of 6 parts N/S e.g. 50ml of concentrate with a maximum of 300ml N/S. Prime giving set fully before commencing infusion. Alternatively the concentrate may be administered undiluted.	See package insert or local policy on epoprostenol in the treatment of peripheral vascular disease.	**Acute Events Which May Accompany Administration** Tachycardia, bradycardia, hypotension, monitor blood pressure and heart rate. A bright redness over the line of vein; exclude infection and treat with a NSAID. Headache, facial flushing, nausea, vomiting, abdominal cramps and jaw pain. Extravasation may cause tissue damage; for management guidelines see section A 7. **pH:** (of diluent) 10.5 **Do not flush** replace giving set. **Sodium content:** 2.5mmol/reconstituted vial. **Displacement:** negligible. **Other comments** Discard any unused infusion after 12 hours. Do not stop infusion for more than a few minutes. **Neonatal information:** Epoprostenol has an antiplatelet effect, therefore heparin should not be added to the infusion bag.	**Incompatible:** do not infuse with other drugs including G and G/S.

Notes

a) For abbreviations used in the table see section A 2.4

b) Prepare a fresh infusion every 24 hours unless otherwise specified.

84

DRUG AND FORMULATION	METHOD	INSTRUCTION FOR DILUTION AND SUITABLE DILUENT	ADMINISTER OVER	COMMENTS	COMPATIBILITY
Ergometrine 500micrograms/1ml	IV bolus.	Dilute with 5ml N/S.	Minimum 1 minute.	**Acute Events Which May Accompany Administration** Nausea and vomiting. Hypertension, bradycardia, palpitations, headache, dizziness and tinnitus may all occur if administered too quickly or undiluted. Extravasation may cause tissue damage; for management guidelines see section A 7. **pH:** 2.7-3.5	
	IM.	Ready diluted.		**Flush:** N/S.	

DRUG AND FORMULATION	METHOD	INSTRUCTION FOR DILUTION AND SUITABLE DILUENT	ADMINISTER OVER	COMMENTS	COMPATIBILITY
Erythromycin Vial 1g	(I) IV infusion.	Reconstitute each 1g with 20ml W to produce 50mg/1ml then further dilute to a maximum concentration of 5mg/1ml with N/S (e.g. 500mg in 100ml). G or G/S may be used instead of N/S, but add 5ml sodium bicarbonate 8.4%/litre of diluent as a buffer.	20-60 minutes.	**Acute Events Which May Accompany Administration** IV infusion may cause thrombophlebitis, check injection site. Arrhythmias may occur when administered as described for fluid restricted patients; cardiac monitoring is required. **pH:** 6.5-7.5 (reconstituted vial) **Flush:** N/S. **Sodium content:** nil. **Displacement:** is allowed for. Add 20ml W to 1g vial to give a concentration of 1g in 20ml (50mg in 1ml).	**Y-site compatible (but see section A 2.6):** aciclovir, aminophylline, magnesium sulphate. **Incompatible:** fluconazole, heparin, gentamicin and all other solutions of pH less than 5.5.
	(C) IV infusion.	Reconstitute as above then dilute as above to a maximum concentration of 1mg/1ml.		**Other comments** Prepare a fresh infusion every 8 hours.	
	(I) IV infusion via a central line for fluid restricted patients (unlicensed).	Reconstitute each 1g with 20ml W to produce 50mg/1ml then dilute 1g to 100ml with N/S.	Minimum 60 minutes.		

Notes

a) For abbreviations used in the table see section A 2.4

b) Prepare a fresh infusion every 24 hours unless otherwise specified.

DRUG AND FORMULATION	METHOD	INSTRUCTION FOR DILUTION AND SUITABLE DILUENT	ADMINISTER OVER	COMMENTS	COMPATIBILITY
Etomidate Ampoule 20mg/10ml	IV bolus into large vein.	May be diluted with N/S or G.	Minimum 2 minutes.	<u>**Acute Events Which May Accompany Administration**</u> There is a high incidence of muscle movement and pain on injection. Pain is reduced if a large vein is used. Diazepam or an opioid analgesic will reduce muscle movement. Hypotension can occur if given too quickly. <u>**pH:**</u> 4-7 <u>**Flush:**</u> N/S or G.	
Fentanyl Ampoule 100microgram/1ml, 500micrograms/ 10ml	IV bolus.	May be diluted with N/S, G, G/S or H.	1-2 minutes.	<u>**Acute Events Which May Accompany Administration**</u> Muscular rigidity may occur with rapid injection. Severe respiratory depression, apnoea, peripheral circulatory collapse, chest wall rigidity, cardiac arrest and anaphylactic shock. Transient hypotension may occur especially in hypovolaemic patients. Monitor blood pressure, heart and respiratory rate. Extravasation may cause tissue damage: for management guidelines see section A 7.	<u>**Y-site compatible (but see section A 2.6):**</u> atracurium, droperidol, heparin, midazolam, mivacurium, pancuronium, potassium chloride, propofol, sodium bicarbonate. **Incompatible:** alkaline agents including methohexitone, thiopentone.
	IM.	Ready diluted.		<u>**pH:**</u> 3.3-6.3 <u>**Flush:**</u> N/S. **Sodium content:** 0.3mmol/1ml.	

DRUG AND FORMULATION	METHOD	INSTRUCTION FOR DILUTION AND SUITABLE DILUENT	ADMINISTER OVER	COMMENTS	COMPATIBILITY
Filgrastim	S/C.	Ready diluted.		<u>**Acute Events Which May Accompany Administration**</u>	<u>**Incompatible:**</u> N/S.
Vial 300micrograms/1ml (30 million units), 480micrograms/ 1.6ml (48 million units)	(I) IV infusion.	Preferred method of infusion: dilute with G to a minimum concentration of 15micrograms/1ml. If lower concentrations of 2-15micrograms/1ml are required then human serum albumin solution at a concentration of 2mg/1ml should be added to the G before the filgrastim is added. A 4.5% solution of albumin contains 45mg/1ml.	30 minutes.	Pain on injection and erythema are more likely if administered rapidly intravenously. **pH:** 4 <u>**Flush:**</u> G. <u>**Sodium content:**</u> negligible. **Other comments** Filgrastim may be adsorbed to glass and plastic therefore do not dilute to a concentration of less than 2micrograms/1ml.	

Notes

a) For abbreviations used in the table see section A 2.4

b) Prepare a fresh infusion every 24 hours unless otherwise specified.

DRUG AND FORMULATION	METHOD	INSTRUCTION FOR DILUTION AND SUITABLE DILUENT	ADMINISTER OVER	COMMENTS	COMPATIBILITY
Flecainide Ampoule 150mg/15ml	IV bolus **Adults:** Maximum dose 150mg.	May be diluted with G.	Minimum 10 minutes.	**Acute Events Which May Accompany Administration** Arrhythmias, monitor ECG continuously, if bolus doses are given. **pH:** 5-6	**Y-site compatible (but see section A 2.6):** digoxin, H, streptokinase. **Incompatible:** alkaline agents and those containing chloride, phosphate or sulphate ions.
	(I) IV infusion.	May be diluted with G.	Minimum 30 minutes for patients with cardiac failure or ventricular tachycardia.	**Flush:** G. **Other comments** Do not use infusion as route of administration for longer than 24 hours.	
	(C) IV infusion via volumetric infusion pump.	See package insert. Dilute with G. If the diluent is N/S, use at least 500ml to prevent precipitation.			
Flucloxacillin Vial 250mg, 500mg	IV bolus (preferred method).	Reconstitute 250-500mg with 5-10ml and 1g with 15-20ml W. May be diluted with N/S, G or G/S.	3-5 minutes.	**Acute Events Which May Accompany Administration** Anaphylaxis. **pH:** 5-7 (reconstituted)	**Y-site compatible (but see section A 2.6):** aminophylline, diamorphine, digoxin, heparin, potassium chloride, ranitidine. **Incompatible:** aminoglycosides, amiodarone, benzylpenicillin, ciprofloxacin, diazepam, morphine.
	(I) IV infusion.	Reconstitute as above then dilute with N/S, G or G/S to 100ml.	30-60 minutes.	**Flush:** N/S. **Sodium content:** 0.57mmol/250mg. **Displacement:** 0.2ml/250mg. Add 4.8ml of diluent to 250mg vial give a	

DRUG AND FORMULATION	METHOD	INSTRUCTION FOR DILUTION AND SUITABLE DILUENT	ADMINISTER OVER	COMMENTS	COMPATIBILITY
	IM.	Reconstitute 250mg with 1.5ml and 500mg with 2ml W.		concentration of 250mg in 5ml (50mg in 1ml).	
Fluconazole Vial 50mg/25ml, 200mg/100ml	(I) IV infusion.	Ready diluted.	10-20mg/ minute.	**pH:** 4-8 **Flush:** N/S. **Sodium content:** 15mmol/200mg (100ml bottle).	**Y-site compatible (but see section A 2.6):** aciclovir, dexamethasone, folinic acid, foscarnet, ganciclovir, heparin, N/S, metronidazole, potassium chloride in G, sodium bicarbonate 8.4%, vancomycin. **Incompatible:** amphotericin, calcium gluconate, ceftazidime, cefuroxime, erythromycin, frusemide, imipenem.
Flucytosine Infusion bottle 2.5g/250ml	(I) IV infusion.	Ready diluted. Administer via a giving set incorporating a 15 micron filter.	20-40 minutes.	**pH:** 7.4 **Flush:** N/S or G. **Sodium content:** 34.5mmol/250ml. **Other comments** Must be stored between 18 and 25°C, otherwise precipitation of flucytosine may occur. Contact Pharmacy if precipitation is visible. Prolonged storage above 25°C could lead to decomposition of flucytosine to 5-fluorouracil.	**Y-site compatible (but see section A 2.6):** N/S, G, or G/S. **Incompatible:** do not infuse with other drugs.

Notes

a) For abbreviations used in the table see section A 2.4

b) Prepare a fresh infusion every 24 hours unless otherwise specified.

DRUG AND FORMULATION	METHOD	INSTRUCTION FOR DILUTION AND SUITABLE DILUENT	ADMINISTER OVER	COMMENTS	COMPATIBILITY
Flumazenil Ampoule 500micrograms/5ml	IV bolus.	May be diluted with N/S or G.	Minimum 15 seconds.	**Acute Events Which May Accompany Administration** Excessive and/or rapidly injected doses may induce benzodiazepine withdrawal symptoms. Transient increases in blood pressure, flushing and rarely seizures especially in epileptic patients. **pH:** 4	Do not infuse with other drugs.
	(I) IV infusion. via volumetric infusion pump.	As above.	100-400micro-grams/hour.	**Flush:** N/S. **Other comments** (I) IV infusion may be useful if drowsiness recurs after IV bolus.	
Folic acid Ampoule 15mg/1ml	IV bolus.	May be diluted with a small volume of N/S e.g. 10ml.	3-5 minutes.	**Acute Events Which May Accompany Administration** Extravasation may cause tissue damage; for management guidelines see section A 7. **pH:** 8-11	**Incompatible:** Will precipitate at pH below 4.5-5.
	IM.	Ready diluted.		**Flush:** N/S.	

DRUG AND FORMULATION	METHOD	INSTRUCTION FOR DILUTION AND SUITABLE DILUENT	ADMINISTER OVER	COMMENTS	COMPATIBILITY
Folinic acid Vial 15mg, 30mg, 350mg/35ml	IV bolus or (I) IV infusion.	Reconstitute 15mg and 30mg vial with 3ml W. For IV infusion dilute with a suitable volume of N/S or G.	Maximum rate 160mg/minute (350mg over at least 3–5 minutes).	**Acute Events Which May Accompany Administration** Hypotension, vasomotor collapse, nausea, vomiting, hot flushes, and sweating may occur if administered too rapidly because of the calcium content. **pH:** 7.7–8.1 **Flush:** N/S. **Sodium content:** 0.2mmol/15mg, 0.4mmol/30mg, 4.6mmol/350mg solution vial.	**Y-site compatible (but see section A 2.6):** cisplatin, fluorouracil, fluconazole, piperacillin/tazobactam. **Incompatible:** trimetrexate.
	IM.	Reconstitute 15mg and 30mg vial with 3ml W.		**Displacement:** 15mg and 30mg vial negligible. **Other comments** Folinic acid 350mg contains 0.7mmol of calcium therefore administer slowly.	
Foscarnet sodium Infusion bottle 24mg/1ml, 250ml, 500ml	(I) IV infusion. via volumetric infusion pump.	If given peripherally, dilute with N/S or G to at least 12mg/1ml. Local practice is to achieve this dilution by piggybacking 1L of N/S with the dose of foscarnet. If given centrally, can be administered undiluted but additional fluids should be given to reduce the risk of	2 hours (local practice).	**Acute Events Which May Accompany Administration** Pins and needles (parasthesia) due to transient hypocalcaemia . Peripheral administration may lead to local irritation and thrombophlebitis. **pH:** 7.4 (undiluted) **Flush:** N/S or G. **Sodium content:** 15.6mmol/1g. **Other comments** One infusion bottle may be used for two doses if being	**Y-site compatible (but see section A 2.6):** cefuroxime, clindamycin, fluconazole, gentamicin, hydrocortisone sodium succinate, metronidazole. **Incompatible:** aciclovir, amphotericin, digoxin, ganciclovir, vancomycin.

Notes

a) For abbreviations used in the table see section A 2.4

b) Prepare a fresh infusion every 24 hours unless otherwise specified.

DRUG AND FORMULATION	METHOD	INSTRUCTION FOR DILUTION AND SUITABLE DILUENT	ADMINISTER OVER	COMMENTS	COMPATIBILITY
		nephrotoxicity.		given twice daily. If contact occurs it may cause local burning sensation, wash skin with water.	
Frusemide Ampoule 20mg/2ml, 50mg/5ml, 250mg/25ml	IV bolus. (C) IV or (I) IV infusion via an syringe or volumetric infusion pump.	May be diluted with N/S. Dilute with N/S to a convenient volume.	**Adults:** Maximum rate 4mg/minute. **Neonates:** Maximum rate 1mg/10 minutes.	**Acute Events Which May Accompany Administration** Rapid administration may result in hearing disorders such as tinnitus and deafness. Extravasation may cause tissue damage; for management guidelines see section A 7. **pH:** 8.7-9.3 **Flush:** N/S. **Sodium content:** 0.3mmol for 20mg/2ml, 0.7mmol for 50mg/5ml, 1mmol for 250mg/25ml.	**Y-site compatible (but see section A 2.6):** adrenaline, aminophylline, atropine, bumetanide, chlormethiazole, digoxin, glyceryl trinitrate, heparin, hydrocortisone sodium succinate, insulin, lignocaine, magnesium sulphate, potassium chloride, ranitidine. **Incompatible:** amiodarone, amphotericin, bleomycin, ciprofloxacin, diazepam, dobutamine, doxapram, droperidol, fluconazole, gentamicin, isoprenaline, morphine, noradrenaline.
Fusidic acid	See sodium fusidate				

DRUG AND FORMULATION	METHOD	INSTRUCTION FOR DILUTION AND SUITABLE DILUENT	ADMINISTER OVER	COMMENTS	COMPATIBILITY
Ganciclovir Vial 500mg	(I) IV infusion either centrally or via a large peripheral vein with good blood flow.	**Handle as for cytotoxic drugs.** Reconstitute each 500mg with 10ml W. Dilute to a concentration not exceeding 10mg/1ml with N/S or G.	Minimum 60 minutes.	**Acute Events Which May Accompany Administration** Pain on infusion, can cause thrombophlebitis. Extravasation may cause tissue damage; for management guidelines see section A 7. **pH:** 10-11 (reconstituted vial) **Flush:** N/S or G. **Sodium content:** 2mmol/500mg. **Displacement:** 0.29ml/500mg. Add 9.7ml of diluent to 500mg vial give a concentration of 500mg/10ml. **Other comments** Do not refrigerate reconstituted vial as ganciclovir will crystallise out.	<u>**Y-site compatible (but see section A 2.6):**</u> fluconazole. **Incompatible:** foscarnet.
Gelofusine (Succinylated gelatin 4% in N/S) Bottle 500ml	(I) IV infusion. For rapid administration a blood administration set can be used.		Dependent on patients need. **Acute blood loss:** 500ml can be given in 5-10 minutes.	**Acute Events Which May Accompany Administration** Severe anaphylactic reactions may occur. **Flush:** N/S. **pH:** 7.4 **Sodium content:** 77mmol/500ml. **Other comments**	<u>**Y-site compatible (but see section A 2.6):**</u> blood.

Notes

a) For abbreviations used in the table see section A 2.4

b) Prepare a fresh infusion every 24 hours unless otherwise specified.

94

DRUG AND FORMULATION	METHOD	INSTRUCTION FOR DILUTION AND SUITABLE DILUENT	ADMINISTER OVER	COMMENTS	COMPATIBILITY
				When given quickly warm bottle to not more than 37°C if possible. Discard unused bottle once seal has been opened.	
Gentamicin Ampoule 20mg/2ml, 80mg/2ml	(I) IV infusion once daily dosing (7mg/kg).	Dilute with 100ml N/S, G or G/S.	1 hour.	**Acute Events Which May Accompany Administration** Extravasation may cause tissue damage; for management guidelines see section A 7. **pH:** 3-5 **Flush:** N/S. **Sodium content:** negligible. **Other comments** Plasma level monitoring is required.	**Y-site compatible (but see section A 2.6):** atracurium, ciprofloxacin, foscarnet, insulin, labetalol, metronidazole, pancuronium. **Incompatible:** amoxycillin, amphotericin, azlocillin, benzylpenicillin, cephalosporins, co-amoxiclav, erythromycin, flucloxacillin, frusemide, heparin, Elohaes (hetastarch), teicoplanin, trimethoprim.
	IV bolus.	Dilution is not normally necessary but may be diluted with N/S (usually 10-20ml).	2 - 3 minutes.		
	IM.	Ready diluted.			

DRUG AND FORMULATION	METHOD	INSTRUCTION FOR DILUTION AND SUITABLE DILUENT	ADMINISTER OVER	COMMENTS	COMPATIBILITY
Glucagon Vial 1unit (~1mg)	IV bolus.	Reconstitute with diluent provided to a concentration of 1unit/1ml. Do not further dilute. If using more than 2 units reconstitute with W to avoid administration of large amounts of preservative.	3-5 minutes.	**Acute Events Which May Accompany Administration** Hypotension, monitor blood pressure. Extravasation may cause tissue damage; for management guidelines section A 7. **pH:** 2.5-3 **Flush:** G or N/S.	
	(C) IV infusion (unlicensed) for cardiogenic shock following beta-blocker overdose via a syringe or volumetric infusion pump.	Reconstitute vial with diluent provided (if using more than 2 units reconstitute with G to avoid administration of large amounts of preservative). Dilute with G to a convenient volume.	**Adults:** 1-10mg/hour. **Children:** 50micrograms/ kg/hour.		
	IM or S/C.	Reconstitute vial with diluent provided.			

Notes

a) For abbreviations used in the table see section A 2.4

b) Prepare a fresh infusion every 24 hours unless otherwise specified.

DRUG AND FORMULATION	METHOD	INSTRUCTION FOR DILUTION AND SUITABLE DILUENT	ADMINISTER OVER	COMMENTS	COMPATIBILITY
Glucose 5% (0.05g/1ml) - 100ml, 250ml, 500ml, 1000ml 10% (0.1g/1ml) - 500ml, 1000ml 15% (0.15g.1ml) - 500ml	IV bolus.	Glucose infusions may be diluted with W if the concentration required is unavailable.	Usually up to 0.5g/kg/hour will not cause glycosuria. Maximum rate should generally not exceed 0.8g/kg/hour.	**Acute Events Which May Accompany Administration** Hyperglycaemia, monitor blood glucose. Fluid overload and electrolyte dilution in congestive conditions. Infusion too quickly may cause local pain and venous irritation. Extravasation may cause tissue damage; for management guidelines section A 7. **Route** G5% is isotonic with blood and may be infused into a peripheral line. If G10% is administered peripherally use a large vein and preferably alter the injection site daily.	Check under individual drug.
20% (0.2g/1ml) - 500ml	(C) IV or (I) IV infusion.	As above.		Concentrations greater than 20% may cause venous irritation and thrombophlebitis if infused peripherally. Central administration is preferable.	
40% (0.4g/1ml) - 500ml 50% (0.5g/1ml) - 50ml, 500ml	IV bolus 50% peripherally into a large vein. Emergency use only.		When administered rapidly for hypoglycaemia give over 1-2 minutes.	**pH:** 3.5-6.5 **Flush:** G or N/S.	

DRUG AND FORMULATION	METHOD	INSTRUCTION FOR DILUTION AND SUITABLE DILUENT	ADMINISTER OVER	COMMENTS	COMPATIBILITY
Glyceryl trinitrate Ampoule 50mg/10ml	(C) IV infusion. Use a non-PVC giving set and syringe to prevent loss of drug.	Dilute with N/S or G to a usual concentration of 1mg/1ml. Concentrations of up to 4mg/1ml have been used. **Paediatric information:** Dilute 1ml of the 50mg/10ml solution to 50ml with N/S or G to give a concentration of 100micrograms/1ml.	Titrate according to response. Rate control recommended.	<u>**Acute Events Which May Accompany Administration**</u> Hypotension, monitor blood pressure. Tachycardia and paradoxical bradycardia which can lead to syncope and collapse, monitor heart rate. <u>**pH:**</u> 3.5-6.5 <u>**Flush:**</u> N/S.	<u>**Y-site compatible (but see section A 2.6):**</u> aminophylline, amiodarone, atracurium, dobutamine, dopamine, frusemide, heparin, insulin, lignocaine, magnesium sulphate, ranitidine, sodium nitroprusside, streptokinase. <u>**Incompatible:**</u> alteplase, hydralazine.
Glycopyrronium Ampoule 200micrograms/1ml 600micrograms/3ml	IV bolus.	May be diluted with N/S, G/S or G.	Rapidly.	<u>**Acute Events Which May Accompany Administration**</u> Arrhythmias, monitor heart rate. Extravasation may cause tissue damage; for management guidelines see section A 7.	<u>**Y-site compatible (but see section A 2.6):**</u> droperidol, midazolam morphine, neostigmine, pethidine.
	IM or S/C (unlicensed).			<u>**pH:**</u> 2.3-4.3 <u>**Flush:**</u> N/S or G.	<u>**Incompatible:**</u> diazepam, methohexitone, thiopentone, alkaline agents.
	(C) S/C infusion (unlicensed).	May dilute with N/S, G/S or G.		<u>**Sodium content:**</u> 0.15mmol/1ml.	

Notes

a) For abbreviations used in the table see section A 2.4

b) Prepare a fresh infusion every 24 hours unless otherwise specified.

DRUG AND FORMULATION	METHOD	INSTRUCTION FOR DILUTION AND SUITABLE DILUENT	ADMINISTER OVER	COMMENTS	COMPATIBILITY
Glycopyrronium 500micrograms **and Neostigmine** 2.5mg Ampoule 1ml	IV bolus.	May dilute with W or N/S.	1-2ml over 10-30 seconds.	<u>**Acute Events Which May Accompany Administration**</u> Arrhythmias and bradycardia, monitor heart rate. <u>**pH:**</u> 3.4-4.1 <u>**Flush:**</u> N/S or G.	Do not infuse with other drugs.
Gonadorelin Vial 100micrograms (HRF)	IV bolus (for pituitary function test).	Reconstitute the HRF vial 100micrograms with 1ml diluent provided.	Few seconds.	<u>**pH:**</u> HRF 4-8, Fertiral 4-5.5, Lutrelef 4-5 <u>**Flush:**</u> N/S.	
Ampoule 1mg/2ml (Fertiral) Ampoule 3.2mg/10ml (Lutrelef unlicensed)	Pulsatile S/C infusion.	Fertiral brand may be further diluted to a convenient volume with N/S. Lutrelef is ready diluted.	One pulse repeated every 90 minutes over 24 hours.	<u>**Other comments**</u> Fertiral is stable in a pump at body temperature for 4 days.	
Granisetron Ampoule 1mg/1ml, 3mg/3ml	IV bolus.	Dilute each 1mg to 5ml and 3mg to 15ml with N/S.	Minimum 30 seconds.	<u>**pH:**</u> 5-7 <u>**Flush:**</u> N/S. <u>**Sodium content:**</u> 1.17mmol/3mg.	<u>**Y-site compatible (but see section A 2.6):**</u> dexamethasone, mannitol 10%.
		Paediatrics: Dilute appropriate dose to 10-30ml	Minimum 5 minutes.		

DRUG AND FORMULATION	METHOD	INSTRUCTION FOR DILUTION AND SUITABLE DILUENT	ADMINISTER OVER	COMMENTS	COMPATIBILITY
		with N/S, G or G/S.			
	(C) S/C infusion (unlicensed) via syringe pump.	May be used undiluted or diluted with N/S or G.			
Haloperidol lactate Ampoule 5mg/1ml, 10mg/2ml, 20mg/2ml	IV bolus.	May be diluted with N/S (concentration prepared must not exceed 500micrograms in 1ml) or G.	1-2 minutes, longer if possible. Maximum rate 5mg/minute.	**Acute Events Which May Accompany Administration** Rapid administration may cause severe hypotension and tachycardia. Monitor blood pressure and heart rate. Extravasation may cause tissue damage; for management guidelines see section A 7. **pH:** 3-3.8	**Compatibility in syringe pump:** with diamorphine see section A 8 for details. Hyoscine hydrobromide. **Y-site compatible (but see section A 2.6):** G, methotrimeprazine, octreotide.
	IM.	Ready diluted.		**Flush:** N/S or G.	
	S/C (unlicensed) or (C) S/C infusion via syringe pump.	Ready diluted.		**Sodium content:** negligible. **Paediatric information:** Avoid IV administration.	

100

Notes

a) For abbreviations used in the table see section A 2.4

b) Prepare a fresh infusion every 24 hours unless otherwise specified.

DRUG AND FORMULATION	METHOD	INSTRUCTION FOR DILUTION AND SUITABLE DILUENT	ADMINISTER OVER	COMMENTS	COMPATIBILITY
Heparin sodium Ampoule 1,000units/1ml, 5,000units/1ml, 25,000units/1ml, 50units/5ml N/S Infusion bag 500units in 500ml N/S	(C) IV infusion (preferred method) via syringe pump.	Dilute required dose with N/S, G or G/S to a convenient volume (25-50ml is usually used).		**Acute Events Which May Accompany Administration** Skin necrosis contraindicates further use of heparin. **pH:** 5-8 **Flush:** N/S. **Other comments** Calcium or sodium heparin may be used subcutaneously. Inject into the lateral abdominal wall using a 26 gauge needle. Insert needle perpendicularly into a pinched fold of skin. Do not rub site of injection.	**Y-site compatible (but see section A 2.6):** aciclovir, adrenaline, aminophylline, amphotericin, atracurium, atropine, azlocillin, benzylpenicillin, calcium salts cefotaxime, ceftazidime, cefuroxime, chloramphenicol, dexamethasone, digoxin, dopamine, fentanyl, flucloxacillin, fluconazole, frusemide, glyceryl trinitrate, hydralazine, isoprenaline, labetalol, lignocaine, magnesium sulphate, methyldopate, metoclopramide, metronidazole, naloxone, neostigmine, noradrenaline, octreotide, pancuronium, phenylephrine, potassium chloride, procainamide, propranolol, ranitidine, streptokinase, suxamethonium, tranexamic acid,
	IV bolus.	Ready diluted.	3-5 minutes.		

DRUG AND FORMULATION	METHOD	INSTRUCTION FOR DILUTION AND SUITABLE DILUENT	ADMINISTER OVER	COMMENTS	COMPATIBILITY
					trimetaphan, urokinase.
Heparin calcium Prefilled syringe 5,000units/0.2ml, 20,000units/0.8ml	S/C.				**Incompatible:** alteplase, amiodarone, desferrioxamine, diazepam, droperidol, methotrimeprazine, opioid analgesics, phenothiazines
Hydralazine Ampoule 20mg	Slow IV bolus.	Reconstitute with 1ml W then dilute to 10ml with N/S.	5-10mg over 2-3 minutes, may be repeated after 20-30 minutes.	**Acute Events Which May Accompany Administration** Tachycardia, hypotension, monitor blood pressure and heart rate. Extravasation may cause tissue damage; for management guidelines see section A 7.	**Y-site compatible (but see section A 2.6):** dobutamine, heparin, potassium chloride. **Incompatible:** G, aminophylline, glyceryl trinitrate, hydrocortisone sodium succinate, sulphonamides.
	(C) IV infusion via volumetric pump.	Reconstitute as above then dilute to 500ml with N/S.	**Adults:** Initially 200-300 micrograms/ minute. Maintenance 50-150 micrograms/ minute.	**pH:** 3.5-4.2 **Flush:** N/S. **Sodium content:** nil. **Displacement:** negligible.	
	(C) IV infusion via syringe pump	Reconstitute 3 ampoules with 1ml W each and further dilute to 60ml with NS (local practice).			
	IM (unlicensed).	Reconstitute with 1ml W.			

Notes

a) For abbreviations used in the table see section A 2.4

b) Prepare a fresh infusion every 24 hours unless otherwise specified.

DRUG AND FORMULATION	METHOD	INSTRUCTION FOR DILUTION AND SUITABLE DILUENT	ADMINISTER OVER	COMMENTS	COMPATIBILITY
Hydrocortisone sodium succinate Vial 100mg	IV bolus.	Reconstitute with 2ml W. May be diluted with N/S, G or G/S.	Minimum 1-10 minutes.	**Acute Events Which May Accompany Administration** Hypotension, cyanosis, cardiac arrest, perianal itch. Monitor blood pressure, heart rate, respiration. **pH:** 7-8 **Flush:** N/S, G. **Sodium content:** 0.5mmol/100mg.	<u>**Y-site compatible (but see section A 2.6)**</u>: aciclovir, adrenaline, aminophylline, amphotericin, calcium gluconate, ceftazidime, chloramphenicol, daunorubicin, foscarnet, frusemide, insulin, lignocaine, magnesium sulphate, morphine, paclitaxel, pancuronium, potassium chloride. **Incompatible:** ciprofloxacin, dacarbazine, ephedrine, heparin, hydralazine.
	(I) IV infusion.	Reconstitute as above then dilute to a maximum concentration of 1mg/1ml with N/S, G, or G/S.	20-30 minutes.		
	IM.	Reconstitute with 2ml W.			
Hyoscine butylbromide Ampoule 20mg/1ml	IV bolus.	May be diluted with G or N/S.	10 seconds.	**Acute Events Which May Accompany Administration** Extravasation may cause tissue damage; for management guidelines see section A 7. **pH:** 3.7-5.5 **Flush:** N/S or G.	<u>**Compatibility in syringe pump:**</u> haloperidol, metoclopramide, midazolam. For diamorphine see section A 8 for details.
	IM.	Ready diluted.			<u>**Y-site compatible (but see section A 2.6)**</u>: most aqueous

DRUG AND FORMULATION	METHOD	INSTRUCTION FOR DILUTION AND SUITABLE DILUENT	ADMINISTER OVER	COMMENTS	COMPATIBILITY
				Sodium content: 0.4 mmol/1ml.	radiological contrast media, diamorphine, morphine, pethidine.
	(C) S/C infusion via syringe pump.	May be diluted with G or N/S.			
Hyoscine hydrobromide Ampoule 400microgram/1ml, 600microgram/1ml	IV bolus (unlicensed).	May be diluted with W.		Acute Events Which May Accompany Administration Bradycardia can occur following low doses. Drowsiness leading to coma (CNS stimulation may precede CNS depression). Toxic doses can cause hyperpyrexia, respiratory depression and rapid respiration. Monitor heart rate, temperature, respiration and sedation level. pH: 5-7 Flush: N/S.	Compatibility in syringe pump: with diamorphine section A 8 for details. Haloperidol, metoclopramide(local practice), midazolam. Y-site compatible (but see section A 2.6): methotrimeprazine, octreotide.
	S/C injection or (C) S/C infusion.	Infusion may be diluted with W.			
	IM.	Ready diluted.		Sodium content: negligible.	
Iloprost (unlicensed) Ampoule 100microgram/1ml (100micrograms = 100,000nanograms)	(I) IV infusion via a syringe pump.	Dilute each ampoule with 50ml N/S or G.	Commence at 0.5nanograms/ kg/minute. Increase dose in increments of 0.5nanograms/ kg/minute every 15-30 minutes to a maximum	Acute Events Which May Accompany Administration Hypotension, tachycardia, arrhythmia, extrasystole, nausea and vomiting. Monitor blood pressure and heart rate every 30 minutes. Stop infusion if side effects occur. Wait one hour and recommence at half previous rate. pH: 7.8-8.8 Flush: N/S or G.	Do not infuse with other drugs.

Notes

a) For abbreviations used in the table see section A 2.4

b) Prepare a fresh infusion every 24 hours unless otherwise specified.

DRUG AND FORMULATION	METHOD	INSTRUCTION FOR DILUTION AND SUITABLE DILUENT	ADMINISTER OVER	COMMENTS	COMPATIBILITY
			of 2nanograms/kg/ minute. Usual total duration of infusion is 6 hours.	**Sodium content:** 0.15mmol/ampoule.	
Imipenem with cilastatin Vial 500mg containing imipenem 500mg with cilastatin 500mg	(I) IV infusion.	Reconstitute 500mg with 100ml N/S, G or G/S.	**Adults:** Doses up to 250-500mg over 20-30 minutes. 1g over 40-60 minutes.	**Acute Events Which May Accompany Administration** Erythema, local pain and induration, thrombophlebitis. Slow infusion rate in patients who develop nausea. **pH:** 6.5-7.5 **Flush:** N/S, G or G/S. **Sodium content:** 1.72mmol/vial. **Displacement:** negligible. **Other comments** Stable for 3 hours at room temperature or 24 hours in a refrigerator after reconstitution with specified diluents.	**Y-site compatible (but see section A 2.6):** aciclovir. **Incompatible:** fluconazole, pethidine.

DRUG AND FORMULATION	METHOD	INSTRUCTION FOR DILUTION AND SUITABLE DILUENT	ADMINISTER OVER	COMMENTS	COMPATIBILITY
Immunoglobulin human normal (Alphaglobin) Vial 2.5g/50ml, 5g/100ml, 10g/200ml	(I) IV infusion.	Ready diluted.	Infuse at a rate of 0.01-0.02ml/kg/minute for the first 30 minutes. If the patient does not experience any discomfort the rate may be increased up to 0.07ml/kg/minute and if tolerated subsequent infusions to the same patient may be at the higher rate.	<u>**Acute Events Which May Accompany Administration**</u> Reactions such as chills, nausea, vomiting and a rise in temperature appear to be related to the rate infusion. **pH:** 5-6 **Other comments** Adrenaline should be available for treatment of any acute anaphylactoid reaction. Follow instructions for the rate of administration very carefully.	Do not infuse with other drugs or fluids.

Notes

a) For abbreviations used in the table see section A 2.4

b) Prepare a fresh infusion every 24 hours unless otherwise specified.

DRUG AND FORMULATION	METHOD	INSTRUCTION FOR DILUTION AND SUITABLE DILUENT	ADMINISTER OVER	COMMENTS	COMPATIBILITY
					Do not infuse with other drugs or fluids.
Immunoglobulin human normal (Vigam-S) Vial 2.5g, 5g	(I) IV infusion.	Reconstitute with the W provided (50ml for 2.5g and 100ml for 5g). Swirl the vial, do not shake.	Infuse at a rate of 0.01-0.02ml/kg/minute for the first 30 minutes. If tolerated the rate may be increased up to 0.04ml/kg/minute up to a maximum of 3ml/minute. On subsequent infusions, for those patients who did not experience an adverse effects, the rate may be cautiously increased to 0.07ml/kg/	**Acute Events Which May Accompany Administration** Reactions such as chills, nausea, vomiting and a rise in temperature appear to be related to the rate infusion. **pH:** 6.5 **Flush:** N/S. **Sodium content:** 16mmol/100ml (reconstituted). **Other comments** Adrenaline should be available for treatment of any acute anaphylactoid reaction. Follow instructions for the rate of administration very carefully. Discard unused infusion 2 hours after reconstitution.	

DRUG AND FORMULATION	METHOD	INSTRUCTION FOR DILUTION AND SUITABLE DILUENT	ADMINISTER OVER	COMMENTS	COMPATIBILITY
			minute.		
Indomethacin Vial 1mg	IV bolus (preferred method).	Reconstitute with 1-2ml N/S or W.	5-10 seconds.	<u>**Acute Events Which May Accompany Administration**</u> Monitor for bleeding. **pH:** 6-7.5	<u>**Incompatible:**</u> G. Do not infuse with other drugs.
	(I) IV infusion via syringe pump (unlicensed).	Reconstitute with 1-2ml N/S or W. Further dilution not recommended.	20 minutes.	**Flush:** N/S. **Sodium content:** negligible. **Displacement:** negligible. **Other comments** Discard solution if cloudy.	

Notes

a) For abbreviations used in the table see section A 2.4

b) Prepare a fresh infusion every 24 hours unless otherwise specified.

108

DRUG AND FORMULATION	METHOD	INSTRUCTION FOR DILUTION AND SUITABLE DILUENT	ADMINISTER OVER	COMMENTS	COMPATIBILITY
Insulin neutral (Actrapid human) Vial 100units/ml 10ml Penfill 150units/1.5ml, Pen 300units/3ml	IV bolus.	Ready diluted.	3-5 minutes.	**Acute Events Which May Accompany Administration**	**Y-site compatible (but see section A 2.6):** adrenaline, amiodarone, digoxin, dopamine, frusemide, gentamicin, glyceryl trinitrate, hydrocortisone sodium succinate, lignocaine, magnesium sulphate, metoclopramide, morphine, noradrenaline, pethidine, potassium chloride, streptokinase, terbutaline.
	(C) IV infusion. Syringe pump recommended.	Dilute in syringe with N/S to 1unit/1ml.	Titrate rate to keep blood glucose in the range of 4 to 8mmol/litre.	Hypoglycaemia, monitor blood glucose. **Flush:** N/S or G. **pH:** neutral **Other comments** Loss of drug into bag, plastic syringe or giving set may occur. When adding insulin to bag, ensure insulin is not injected into dead space of injection port of infusion bag.	
	(C) IV infusion via volumetric pump (GKI regimen). Used occasionally in minor elective surgery in diabetic	Typically 10-15 units insulin and 10mmol potassium chloride added to 500ml G10%. The concentration of insulin may be increased or decreased by 2-4units in each 500ml G10% to maintain blood glucose levels in the	100ml/hour.		**Incompatible:** aminophylline, co-trimoxazole and other sulphonamides, octreotide, phenytoin, sodium bicarbonate, thiopentone.

DRUG AND FORMULATION	METHOD	INSTRUCTION FOR DILUTION AND SUITABLE DILUENT	ADMINISTER OVER	COMMENTS	COMPATIBILITY
	patients.	range of 4-8mmol/litre, as clinically indicated.			
	IM or S/C.	Ready diluted.			
Iron hydroxide sucrose complex (Venofer) (Unlicensed) Ampoule 100mg/5ml of elemental iron	(I) IV infusion via volumetric infusion pump.	Dilute dose to 1mg/1ml N/S.	Initial rate: 25ml over the first 15 minutes. Titrate upwards over next 30 minutes according to patient tolerance. Maximum rate: 200ml/hour.	**Acute Events Which May Accompany Administration** Anaphylaxis: have resuscitation equipment available. Administer hydrocortisone 100mg IV and ibuprofen 200mg PO immediately before dose. Phlebitis, extravasation may cause tissue damage. Nursing observations are required every 15 minutes. The higher the dose the greater the risk of side effects. **Flush:** N/S. **Other comments** Do not use ampoules if any sediment is present. A more dilute solution may be used as a result of patient intolerance.	Do not infuse with other drugs.
Isoniazid	IV bolus.	Ready diluted.	3-5 minutes.	**pH:** 5.6-6 **Flush:** N/S.	**Incompatible:** glucose solutions.
	IM.	Ready diluted.			
Isoprenaline Ampoule 2mg/2ml, Min-I-Jet	(C) IV infusion with a volumetric infusion pump	Dilute with G (adults: usually to 500ml).	Adjust rate according to response and indication.	**Acute Events Which May Accompany Administration** May precipitate ventricular extrasystoles and arrythmias. If heart rate >100 beats/minute or if	**Y-site compatible (but see section A 2.6):** amiodarone, atracurium, calcium chloride, dobutamine, heparin, magnesium

Notes

a) For abbreviations used in the table see section A 2.4

b) Prepare a fresh infusion every 24 hours unless otherwise specified.

110

DRUG AND FORMULATION	METHOD	INSTRUCTION FOR DILUTION AND SUITABLE DILUENT	ADMINISTER OVER	COMMENTS	COMPATIBILITY
200micrograms/10ml	preferably via a central line.			premature heart beats or changes in **ECG** develop consider slowing or stopping infusion. Extravasation may cause tissue damage; for management guidelines see section A 7. **pH:** 2.5-2.8	sulphate, noradrenaline, pancuronium, potassium chloride. **Incompatible:** frusemide, sodium bicarbonate.
	IV bolus.	Ready diluted.	3-5 minutes.	**Flush:** G.	
Ketamine Vial 200mg/20ml, 500mg/5ml, 500mg/10ml	IV bolus.	Ready diluted.	Minimum 60 seconds.	**Acute Events Which May Accompany Administration** Temporary elevation of blood pressure and heart rate frequently occur (~25% increase in baseline blood pressure). Also arrhythmias, laryngospasm, respiratory depression and hypotension.	**Compatibility in syringe pump:** with diamorphine section A 8 for details. Also compatible with lignocaine (local practice).
	(C) IV infusion via volumetric infusion or syringe pump.	Dilute to 1mg/1ml with G or N/S. In fluid restriction dilute to a maximum concentration of 50mg/1ml (unlicensed).	Dependent on indication, see package insert for details.	Tonic and clonic movements resembling seizures may occur and are not an indication for adjusting therapy. Extravasation may cause tissue damage; for management guidelines see section A 7. **pH:** 3.5-5.5	**Y-site compatible (but see section A 2.6):** midazolam, morphine. **Incompatible:** barbiturates, doxapram.
	(C) SC infusion via syringe pump (unlicensed).	Dilute with N/S.		**Flush:** N/S or G. **Sodium content:** negligible.	
Ketorolac Ampoule 10mg/1ml	IV bolus.	May be diluted with N/S or G.	Minimum 15 seconds.	**Acute Events Which May Accompany Administration** Anaphylaxis, bradycardia and flushing. Monitor blood pressure and heart rate.	**Compatibility in syringe pump:** with diamorphine see section A 8 for details.
	IM.	Ready diluted.		**pH:** 6.9-7.9 **Flush:** N/S or G.	**Incompatible:** morphine, pethidine, promethazine.

DRUG AND FORMULATION	METHOD	INSTRUCTION FOR DILUTION AND SUITABLE DILUENT	ADMINISTER OVER	COMMENTS	COMPATIBILITY
	(C) S/C infusion via syringe pump (unlicensed).	May be diluted with W.		**Other comments** Only licensed for use on up to 2 consecutive days.	
Labetalol Ampoule 100mg/20ml	IV bolus.	Ready diluted.	Maximum rate 50mg/minute can be repeated every 5 minutes to a maximum dose of 200mg.	**Acute Events Which May Accompany Administration** Bradycardia, monitor of **ECG** recommended. Hypotension, monitor blood pressure; the patient should remain supine for more than 3 hours after administration. Extravasation may cause tissue damage; for management guidelines see section A 7. **pH:** 3.5-4.2 **Flush:** N/S. **Sodium content:** negligible.	**Y-site compatible (but see section A 2.6):** dopamine, gentamicin, heparin, magnesium sulphate, morphine, pethidine, potassium chloride, ranitidine. **Incompatible:** sodium bicarbonate.
	(C) IV infusion via volumetric infusion.	Dilute to 1mg/1ml with G/S or G.	Usual maximum rate 2mg/minute.		
Lenograstim Vial 105micrograms (13.4MU), 263micrograms (33.6MU)	SC.	Reconstitute each vial with 1ml W provided. Mix gently until dissolved. Do not shake vigorously.		**Acute Events Which May Accompany Administration** Pain at injection site when given SC. More likely to occur if vial is taken straight out of fridge prior to administration.	
	(I) IV infusion.	Reconstitute as above and further dilute in N/S to a final concentration of not less than 2micrograms/1ml for 105micrograms vial and 2.5micrograms/1ml for the	30 minutes	**pH:** 6.5 **Flush:** N/S. **Sodium content:** negligible.	

Notes

a) For abbreviations used in the table see section A 2.4

b) Prepare a fresh infusion every 24 hours unless otherwise specified.

DRUG AND FORMULATION	METHOD	INSTRUCTION FOR DILUTION AND SUITABLE DILUENT	ADMINISTER OVER	COMMENTS	COMPATIBILITY
		263micrograms vial.			**Y-site compatible (but see section A 2.6):** adrenaline, alteplase, aminophylline, amiodarone, bretylium, calcium chloride, calcium gluconate, ciprofloxacin, digoxin, dopamine, dobutamine, frusemide, glyceryl trinitrate, heparin, hydrocortisone sodium succinate, insulin, morphine noradrenaline, phenylephrine, potassium chloride, procainamide, sodium nitroprusside, streptokinase. **Incompatible:** phenytoin.
Lignocaine Min-I-Jet 1% (100mg/10ml) Infusion bag 0.1% (1mg/ml), 0.2% (2mg/ml), 0.4% (4mg/ml) in G 500ml Ampoule 0.5% (100mg/20ml)	IV bolus (initial loading dose followed by infusion).		**Adults:** Usual maximum rate 50mg/minute.	**Acute Events Which May Accompany Administration** Rapid administration may produce dizziness, paraesthesia and drowsiness. Hypotension and tachycardia leading to arrest, **ECG** monitoring required. CNS and peripheral reactions are dose related. Extravasation may cause tissue damage; for management guidelines see section A 7. **pH:** 3.5-6 (pre-mixed infusion), 5-7 (Min-I-Jet) **Flush:** N/S. **Sodium content:** variable.	
1% (20mg/2ml, 50mg/5ml), 2% (40mg/2ml, 100mg/5ml, 400mg/20ml)	(C) IV infusion via volumetric infusion pump.	Dilute with G or N/S to suggested concentration of 0.1-0.4%. Use ready prepared solutions where possible.	**Adults:** Maximum rate 4mg/minute.		
Liothyronine Ampoule	IV bolus.	Reconstitute with 1-2ml W.	3-5 minutes.	**Acute Events Which May Accompany Administration** Arrhythmias, tachycardia, palpitation and cramp in skeletal muscle, monitor pulse.	

DRUG AND FORMULATION	METHOD	INSTRUCTION FOR DILUTION AND SUITABLE DILUENT	ADMINISTER OVER	COMMENTS	COMPATIBILITY
20micrograms				Extravasation may cause tissue damage; for management guidelines see section A 7. **pH:** 11 **Flush:** N/S. **Sodium content:** negligible.	
Lorazepam Ampoule 4mg/1ml	IV bolus. Avoid injecting into small veins.	May be diluted up to 2ml with N/S or W.	Usually 3-5 minutes. Maximum rate 2mg/minute.	<u>**Acute Events Which May Accompany Administration**</u> Rapid administration increases risk of respiratory depression and hypotension. Monitor blood pressure and respiratory rate.	**Incompatible:** buprenorphine,
	IM.	Dilute up to 2ml with N/S or W.		**pH:** Non-aqueous solution therefore no pH. **Flush:** N/S.	

Notes

a) For abbreviations used in the table see section A 2.4

b) Prepare a fresh infusion every 24 hours unless otherwise specified.

DRUG AND FORMULATION	METHOD	INSTRUCTION FOR DILUTION AND SUITABLE DILUENT	ADMINISTER OVER	COMMENTS	COMPATIBLITY
Magnesium sulphate Ampoule 50% 1g/2ml, 5g/10ml containing 2.03mmol Mg^{2+}/1ml	IV bolus.	Dilute to a maximum concentration of 200mg/1ml with N/S or G.	3-5 minutes. **Adults:** Maximum rate 150mg/minute.	**Acute Events Which May Accompany Administration** Rapid administration may cause flushing and hypotension. In pregnancy blood pressure, respiratory rate, magnesium plasma levels and fluid monitoring is necessary and **ECG** monitoring recommended. Extravasation may cause tissue damage; for management guidelines see section A 7. **pH:** 5.5-8 **Flush:** N/S.	<u>Y-site compatible (but see section A 2.6):</u> amphotericin, calcium gluconate, chlormethiazole, co-trimoxazole, dobutamine, erythromycin, frusemide, glyceryl trinitrate, heparin, hydrocortisone sodium succinate, insulin, isoprenaline, labetalol, methyldopate, metronidazole, morphine, noradrenaline, potassium chloride, streptokinase. **Incompatible:** alkaline agents, clindamycin, sulphates.
	(1) IV infusion.	Dilute each 1g (4mmol magnesium) to a suitable volume (at least 10ml) with N/S or G.	**Adults:** Usual dose 1-2g/hour.		
	IM in alternate buttocks.	Adult doses may be diluted to 25%. Paediatric doses must be diluted to 20% in G or N/S.			

DRUG AND FORMULATION	METHOD	INSTRUCTION FOR DILUTION AND SUITABLE DILUENT	ADMINISTER OVER	COMMENTS	COMPATIBILITY
Mannitol Infusion bag 10% (0.1g/1ml), 20% (0.2g/1ml), 500ml	IV bolus - test dose.	Ready diluted.	0.2g/kg over 3-5 minutes.	**Acute Events Which May Accompany Administration** Nausea, vomiting, thirst, headache, chills, fever, tachycardia, chest pain, hypo or hypertension. Extravasation may cause tissue damage; for management guidelines see section A 7. **pH:** 4.5-7 **Flush:** N/S or G.	**Y-site compatible (but see section A 2.6):** chlormethiazole, cisplatin, fluorouracil, dopamine, granisetron, ondansetron, paclitaxel, potassium chloride (local practice). **Incompatible:** in strongly alkaline or acidic solutions.
	(I) IV infusion via volumetric infusion pump preferably centrally.	Ready diluted.	**Adults:** 1-2g/kg over 30-60 minutes.	**Other comments** Central administration is preferred because extravasation can cause oedema, skin necrosis and thrombophlebitis. Use administration sets incorporating a filter for concentrations of 20%. Infusion may crystallise at low temperatures; redissolve by warming.	
Meropenem Vial 250mg, 500mg, 1g	IV bolus.	Reconstitute each 250mg with W 5ml. This produces an approximate concentration of 50mg/1ml.	5 minutes.	**Acute Events Which May Accompany Administration** Thrombophlebitis and rash. **pH:** 7.3-8.3	Do not infuse with other drugs.
	(I) IV infusion.	Reconstitute as above and	15-30 minutes.	**Flush:** N/S or G.	

Notes

a) For abbreviations used in the table see section A 2.4

b) Prepare a fresh infusion every 24 hours unless otherwise specified.

DRUG AND FORMULATION	METHOD	INSTRUCTION FOR DILUTION AND SUITABLE DILUENT	ADMINISTER OVER	COMMENTS	COMPATIBILITY
		further dilute dose to 50-250ml with N/S or G.		**Sodium content:** 3.9mmol per 1g. **Displacement:** 0.2ml/250mg. Add 4.8ml W to 250mg vial to give a concentration of 50mg/1ml.	
Mesna Ampoule 400mg/4ml, 1000mg/10ml	(I) IV infusion.	Dilute with a convenient volume of N/S or G.	15-30 minutes.	**Acute Events Which May Accompany Administration** Nausea, vomiting, diarrhoea, fatigue, rash, hypotension, tachycardia.	**Compatible in infusion bag (but see section A 2.6):** cyclophosphamide, ifosfamide, potassium chloride.
	IV bolus.	Ready diluted.	3 minutes	**pH:** 6.5-8.5 **Flush:** N/S.	**Incompatible:** carboplatin, cisplatin.
	(C) IV infusion via volumetric infusion pump following an (I) IV loading dose.	Dilute with a convenient volume of N/S or G.	30 minutes - 24 hours.		
Methohexitone sodium Vial 100mg, 500mg	IV bolus.	Reconstitute with W, N/S or G. Add 10ml to 100mg vial and 50ml to 500mg vial.	10mg/5 seconds.	**Acute Events Which May Accompany Administration** Temporary hypotension and tachycardia may occur, monitor blood pressure and heart rate. Extravasation may cause tissue damage; for management guidelines see section A 7. **pH:** 10-11 (1% solution)	**Incompatible:** do not infuse with other drugs.

DRUG AND FORMULATION	METHOD	INSTRUCTION FOR DILUTION AND SUITABLE DILUENT	ADMINISTER OVER	COMMENTS	COMPATIBILITY
				Flush: N/S or G.	
Metho-trimeprazine Ampoule 25mg/1ml	IV bolus.	Dilute with at least an equal volume of N/S before administration.	3-5 minutes.	**Acute Events Which May Accompany Administration** Postural hypotension particularly in patients over 50, monitor blood pressure. **Other comments** Discard infusion if pink or yellow colouration occurs. **pH:** 4.5	**Compatibility in syringe pump:** with diamorphine see section A 8 for details. **Y-site compatible (but see section A 2.6):** diamorphine, hyoscine hydrobromide, haloperidol, metoclopramide.
	IM.	Ready diluted.		**Flush:** N/S. **Sodium content:** negligible.	**Incompatible:** alkaline agents, heparin, ranitidine.
	(C) S/C via syringe pump.	Dilute with a suitable volume of W (local practice) or N/S.			

Notes

a) For abbreviations used in the table see section A 2.4

b) Prepare a fresh infusion every 24 hours unless otherwise specified.

118

DRUG AND FORMULATION	METHOD	INSTRUCTION FOR DILUTION AND SUITABLE DILUENT	ADMINISTER OVER	COMMENTS	COMPATIBILITY
Methoxamine Ampoule 20mg/1ml	IV bolus - Emergency use into a large vein.	Ready diluted.	1mg/minute.	**Acute Events Which May Accompany Administration** Hypertension may occur if infused too quickly. In previously normotensive patients, systolic blood pressure should be maintained at 80-100mmHg. In previously hypertensive patients, systolic blood pressure should be maintained at 30-40 mmHg below normal. Extravasation may cause tissue damage; for management guidelines see section A 7.	Do not infuse with other drugs.
	(C) IV infusion via a volumetric infusion pump (unlicensed). See above for route.	Dilute with 250ml G or N/S.		If extravasation occurs infiltrate as soon as possible with 10-15ml of N/S containing 5-10mg phentolamine to prevent slough and necrosis.Use a fine needle and infiltrate liberally throughout the ischaemic area. **pH:** 4.4 **Flush:** N/S or G. **Sodium content:** negligible.	
	IM.	Ready diluted.			
Methyldopate	(I) IV infusion. via a volumetric infusion pump.	Dilute to 100ml with G.	30-60 minutes.	**Acute Events Which May Accompany Administration** Paradoxical hypertensive response, monitor blood	**Y-site compatible (but see section A 2.6):** heparin, magnesium sulphate, morphine,

DRUG AND FORMULATION	METHOD	INSTRUCTION FOR DILUTION AND SUITABLE DILUENT	ADMINISTER OVER	COMMENTS	COMPATIBILITY
Ampoule 250mg/5ml				pressure. Extravasation may cause tissue damage; for management guidelines section A 7. **pH:** 3-4.2 **Flush:** N/S or G. **Sodium content:** negligible.	potassium chloride. **Incompatible:** amphotericin.
Methylene Blue Ampoule 1 % 5ml	IV bolus (unlicensed) used in hypotension associated with sepsis and methaemaglo-binaemia.	Ready diluted.	Several minutes (as slow as possible).	**Acute Events Which May Accompany Administration** Hypertension, monitor blood pressure. Rapid injection may produce additional methaemoglobinaemia. Extravasation may cause tissue damage; for management guidelines section A 7. **pH:** 3-4.5 **Flush:** N/S	
	(C) IV infusion (unlicensed) for methaemaglo-binaemia.	Dilute in G/S to a convenient volume.	Suggested 1-2mg/kg bolus followed by 0.1-0.15mg/kg/hour.	**Sodium content:** nil.	
Methyl-prednisolone sodium succinate Vial 40mg, 125mg, 500mg, 1g, 2g	IV bolus (doses less than 250mg).	Reconstitute with diluent provided.	Give slowly minimum 5 minutes.	**Acute Events Which May Accompany Administration** Bradycardia and rarely anaphylaxis. If administered too quickly cardiac arrhythmias, circulatory collapse and cardiac arrest may occur.	**Y-site compatible (but see section A 2.6):** Hep/S. **Incompatible:** ciprofloxacin, potassium chloride.
	(I) IV infusion (doses over	Reconstitute as above then further dilute with G, N/S or	Minimum 30 minutes.	**pH:** 7.4-8	

Notes

a) For abbreviations used in the table see section A 2.4

b) Prepare a fresh infusion every 24 hours unless otherwise specified.

DRUG AND FORMULATION	METHOD	INSTRUCTION FOR DILUTION AND SUITABLE DILUENT	ADMINISTER OVER	COMMENTS	COMPATIBILITY
	250mg).	G/S.		**Flush:** N/S, G. **Sodium content:** 2mmol/g. **Other comments** Use infusion within 6 hours. Inspect for particulate matter or discolouration prior to administration.	
	IM (for doses up to 40mg).	Reconstitute with diluent provided.			
Metoclopramide Ampoule 10mg/2ml	IV bolus.	May be diluted with N/S (usually 10-20ml).	1-2 minutes.	**Acute Events Which May Accompany Administration** Dystonic reactions, particularly in children and young women. **pH:** 10mg/2ml = 3-5. 100mg/20ml = 5-7. **Flush:** N/S or G. **Sodium content:** 10mg/2ml negligible, 100mg/20ml = 2.74mmol.	**Compatibility in syringe pump:** with diamorphine see section A 8 for details. Haloperidol, heparin, hyoscine butylbromide, hyoscine hydrobromide (local practice), insulin, methotrimeprazine, morphine. **Y-site compatible (but see section A 2.6):** dexamethasone, droperidol, heparin, insulin, methotrimeprazine.
	IM.	Ready diluted.			
	S/C bolus or (C) S/C infusion (widespread practice).	Ready diluted. May be further diluted with W or N/S.			
Metoclopramide Ampoule 100mg/20ml	(C) IV infusion (preferred method).	Loading dose 2-4mg/kg in 50-100ml N/S, G, G/S or H. Maintenance 3-5mg/kg in 500ml diluent.	Loading dose 15-30 minutes. Maintenance 8-12 hours.		
	(I) IV infusion.	Up to 2mg/kg in a minimum of 50ml N/S, G, G/S or H.	Minimum 15 minutes.		

DRUG AND FORMULATION	METHOD	INSTRUCTION FOR DILUTION AND SUITABLE DILUENT	ADMINISTER OVER	COMMENTS	COMPATIBILITY
Metronidazole Infusion bag 500mg/100ml Ampoule 100mg/20ml	(I) IV infusion.	Infusion bag is ready diluted. Ampoules may be further diluted with N/S, G/S or G.	**Adults:** 25mg/minute (i.e. 500mg over 20 minutes). **Children:** 20 minutes.	**pH:** 5.5-5.7 **Flush:** N/S, G or G/S. **Sodium content:** 2.7mmol/100mg ampoule, 13.15mmol/500mg infusion.	Any one of amikacin, ceftazidime, cefotaxime and cefuroxime may be added to an infusion of metronidazole. **Y-site compatible (but see section A 2.6):** aciclovir, aminophylline, amiodarone, amoxycillin, azlocillin, chlormethiazole, ciprofloxacin, dexamethasone, fluconazole, foscarnet, gentamicin, heparin, magnesium sulphate, morphine, potassium chloride, tobramycin. **Incompatible:** G10%, H, azlocillin, trimethoprim.
Metoprolol Ampoule 5mg/5ml	IV bolus.	May be diluted with N/S or G.	1-2mg/minute.	**Acute Events Which May Accompany Administration** Hypotension, bradycardia and cardiac arrhythmias. Monitor blood pressure and heart rate. **pH:** 5.5-7.5 **Flush:** N/S. **Sodium content:** 0.8mmol/ampoule.	

Notes

a) For abbreviations used in the table see section A 2.4
b) Prepare a fresh infusion every 24 hours unless otherwise specified.

DRUG AND FORMULATION	METHOD	INSTRUCTION FOR DILUTION AND SUITABLE DILUENT	ADMINISTER OVER	COMMENTS	COMPATIBILITY
Mexiletine Ampoule 250mg/10ml	IV bolus (loading dose).	Ready diluted.	25mg/minute.	**Acute Events Which May Accompany Administration** Hypotension, monitor blood pressure. Sinus bradycardia, atrial fibrillation, atrioventricular dissociation and exacerbation of arrhythmias.	
	(C) IV infusion (additional loading dose and maintenance dose).	See package insert for details. Dilute with 250-500ml N/S or G.	See package insert for details.	Monitor **ECG**. **pH:** 5-6 **Flush:** N/S or G.	
Midazolam Ampoule 10mg/2ml, 10mg/5ml	IV bolus.	Ready diluted.	30 seconds minimum. Usually given over 2 minutes and repeated at intervals of at least 2 minutes.	**Acute Events Which May Accompany Administration** Respiratory depression and arrest have occurred when doses are given too quickly. Extravasation may cause tissue damage; for management guidelines see section A 7. **pH:** 3 (approximately)	**Compatibility in syringe pump:** with diamorphine see section A 8 for details. Hyoscine hydrobromide. **Y-site compatible (but see section A 2.6):** alfentanil, atracurium, atropine, droperidol, fentanyl, glycopyrronium, hyoscine butylbromide, ketamine, mivacurium, morphine, octreotide, pancuronium.
	(C) IV infusion via syringe pump following initial loading	Dilute if required with N/S, G or G/S.		**Flush:** N/S. **Sodium content:** negligible.	

DRUG AND FORMULATION	METHOD	INSTRUCTION FOR DILUTION AND SUITABLE DILUENT	ADMINISTER OVER	COMMENTS	COMPATIBILITY
	dose over 5 minutes.				**Incompatible:** ranitidine.
	(C) S/C infusion via syringe pump (unlicensed).	Dilute with W.			
Mivacurium Ampoule 10mg/5ml, 20mg/10ml	IV bolus.	May be administered undiluted, or diluted with N/S, G or G/S to a concentration of 500micrograms/1ml.	5-15 seconds but see 'Other comments'.	**Acute Events Which May Accompany Administration** Hypotension, monitor blood pressure. **pH:** 4.5 **Flush:** N/S. **Sodium content:** negligible. **Other comments** Doses up to 150micrograms/kg may be given over 5-15 seconds, higher doses should be given over 30	**Y-site compatible (but see section A 2.6):** alfentanil, droperidol, fentanyl, midazolam. **Incompatible:** alkaline agents e.g. thiopentone.
	(C) IV infusion.	As above.	8-10 micrograms/kg/minute adjusted according to patient response.	seconds. Give IV bolus over 60 seconds to patients with cardiovascular disease, those with increased sensitivity to histamine and those who may be unusually sensitive to falls in blood pressure.	

Notes

a) For abbreviations used in the table see section A 2.4

b) Prepare a fresh infusion every 24 hours unless otherwise specified.

DRUG AND FORMULATION	METHOD	INSTRUCTION FOR DILUTION AND SUITABLE DILUENT	ADMINISTER OVER	COMMENTS	COMPATIBILITY
Morphine Ampoule 10mg/1ml, 30mg/1ml	IV bolus.	May be diluted with N/S, G, G10% or G/S.	3-5 minutes.	**Acute Events Which May Accompany Administration** Severe respiratory depression, apnoea, hypotension, peripheral circulatory collapse, chest wall rigidity, cardiac arrest and anaphylactic shock. Monitor blood pressure, heart and respiratory rate. Extravasation may cause tissue damage; for management guidelines see section A 7. **pH:** 2.5-4.5 **Flush:** N/S, G or G/S. **Sodium content:** negligible. **Other comments** Repeated S/C injections may cause local irritation, pain and induration.	**Compatibility in syringe pump:** Morphine 1mg/1ml and cyclizine <2mg/1ml in N/S (local practice), metoclopramide. **Y-site compatible (but see section A 2.6):** atracurium, atropine, cefuroxime, co-trimoxazole, cyclizine (local practice), dexamethasone, digoxin, droperidol, glycopyrronium, hydrocortisone sodium succinate, hyoscine butylbromide, insulin, ketamine, labetalol, lignocaine, magnesium sulphate, methyldopate, metoclopramide, metronidazole, midazolam, pancuronium, potassium chloride, propofol (local practice), propranolol, suxamethonium, vancomycin. **Incompatible:** aciclovir, alkaline agents, aminophylline, flucloxacillin, frusemide, heparin,
	(C) IV infusion or (C) S/C infusion	Dilute in N/S or G usually to 1mg/1ml.			

DRUG AND FORMULATION	METHOD	INSTRUCTION FOR DILUTION AND SUITABLE DILUENT	ADMINISTER OVER	COMMENTS	COMPATIBILITY
	(unlicensed) via syringe pump.				ketorolac, phenytoin, sodium bicarbonate, thiopentone.
	IM or S/C. See 'Other comments'.	Ready diluted.			
Muromonab-CD3 (OKT3) (unlicensed) Ampoule 5mg/5ml	IV bolus.	Ready diluted.	30-60 seconds.	<u>**Acute Events Which May Accompany Administration**</u> Initially fever and chills followed by dyspnoea, tremor, chest pain/tightness, wheezing, diarrhoea, nausea and vomiting, tachycardia, hyper and hypotension, joint pain, pruritis and rash. Facilities for CPR and monitoring are necessary. **pH:** 7 **Other comments** Methylprednisolone 8mg/kg IV 1-4 hours before OKT3 administration is strongly recommended. Alternatively hydrocortisone 100mg IV 30 minutes prior to dose may be given. Do not shake vial. OKT3 solution may develop fine translucent particles which do not affect potency.	Do not administer with other drugs.

Notes

a) For abbreviations used in the table see section A 2.4

b) Prepare a fresh infusion every 24 hours unless otherwise specified.

DRUG AND FORMULATION	METHOD	INSTRUCTION FOR DILUTION AND SUITABLE DILUENT	ADMINISTER OVER	COMMENTS	COMPATIBILITY
Naloxone Ampoule 40micrograms/2ml, 400micrograms/1ml	IV bolus.	The 400micrograms/1ml solution may be diluted with W or N/S immediately before use to a concentration of 20micrograms/1ml.		**Acute Events Which May Accompany Administration** Hypotension, hypertension, ventricular tachycardia and fibrillation. Precipitation of acute withdrawal syndrome. Extravasation may cause tissue damage; for management guidelines see section A 7. **pH:** 3-4.5	<u>**Y-site compatible (but see section A 2.6):**</u> chlormethiazole, heparin. **Incompatible:** alkaline agents.
	(C) or (I) IV infusion via syringe or volumetric infusion pump.	Dilute with G, G/S or N/S to 4micrograms/1ml.	According to response.	**Flush:** N/S or G. **Sodium content:** negligible. **Other comments** Use infusion within 12 hours. Inspect infusion solutions for particulate matter and discolouration before administration.	
	IM or S/C.	Ready diluted.			
Neostigmine Ampoule 2.5mg/1ml	IV bolus.	May be diluted with W immediately before use.	Minimum 3-5 minutes.	**Acute Events Which May Accompany Administration** Abdominal cramps, diarrhoea, salivation. **pH:** 4.5-6.5 **Flush:** N/S. **Sodium content:** negligible. **Other comments**	<u>**Y-site compatible (but see section A 2.6):**</u> heparin, glycopyrronium, potassium chloride.

DRUG AND FORMULATION	METHOD	INSTRUCTION FOR DILUTION AND SUITABLE DILUENT	ADMINISTER OVER	COMMENTS	COMPATIBILITY
				Have atropine available to counteract possible cholinergic reactions.	
	IM or S/C.	Ready diluted.			
Nimodipine Vial 10mg/50ml (0.02%)	(I) IV infusion Must be administered centrally via a syringe pump connected to a 3 way tap into a running drip (40ml/hour) of either N/S or G (see data sheet for full details).	Ready diluted.	500micrograms-2mg/hour (see package insert for details).	**Acute Events Which May Accompany Administration** Hypotension, monitor blood pressure. Tachycardia or bradycardia, monitor heart rate. Flushing can also occur. **pH:** 6-7.5 **Flush:** N/S or G. **Other comments:** Incompatible with PVC; use polyethylene or polypropylene apparatus provided. Protect infusion line and syringe from light.	Do not infuse with other drugs.
Noradrenaline acid tartrate Ampoule 4mg/2ml (equivalent to 2mg/2ml noradrenaline base)	(C) or (I) IV infusion into a central line via a syringe pump.	Standard dilution: 2, 4 or 8mg noradrenaline base/ 50ml G/S or G via a central line (local practice). Higher or lower concentrations may be prepared if necessary.	Adjust rate according to response.	**Acute Events Which May Accompany Administration** Avoid peripheral administration because extravasation can produce local vasoconstriction leading to severe tissue hypoxia and ischaemia; for management guidelines see section A 7. Noradrenaline infusions should only be used in areas where appropriate cardiovascular monitoring is available (ITU, HDU etc). **pH:** 3-4.5 **Do not flush** replace giving set.	**Y-site compatible (but see section A 2.6):** adrenaline, amiodarone, calcium salts, dobutamine, dopamine, heparin, insulin, isoprenaline, lignocaine, magnesium sulphate, potassium chloride. **Incompatible:** aminophylline, frusemide, sodium bicarbonate, thiopentone.

Notes

a) For abbreviations used in the table see section A 2.4

b) Prepare a fresh infusion every 24 hours unless otherwise specified.

128

DRUG AND FORMULATION	METHOD	INSTRUCTION FOR DILUTION AND SUITABLE DILUENT	ADMINISTER OVER	COMMENTS	COMPATIBILITY
				Other comments pH of diluent must be below 6. Loss of potency occurs if diluent is N/S. Discard infusion if brown colour develops. 1:1000 solution contains 1mg noradrenaline base/1ml.	
Octreotide Ampoule 50micrograms/1ml, 100micrograms/1ml 500micrograms/1ml	S/C (preferred method).	Dilution is not required.		**Acute Events Which May Accompany Administration** Bradycardia, hypotension, facial flushing, hyperglycaemia and rarely hypoglycaemia. Monitor cardiac rhythms, **ECG**, blood glucose, blood pressure and heart rate with IV doses. Extravasation may cause tissue damage; for management guidelines see section A 7.	**Compatibility in syringe pump:** with diamorphine see section A 8 for details. **Y-site compatible (but see section A 2.6):** haloperidol, heparin, hyoscine hydrobromide, midazolam.
	IV bolus.	Dilute dose with N/S to a ratio of not less than 1:1 and not more than 1:9 by volume.	3-5 minutes.	Rapid administration of the IV bolus may produce stinging at the injection site and a brief drop in heart rate.	**Incompatible:** cyclizine, G, insulin, steroids.
	(C) S/C infusion (unlicensed) via syringe pump.	Dilute dose to a suitable volume with N/S (local practice).		**pH:** 3.9-4.5 **Flush:** N/S. **Sodium content:** negligible. **Other comments**	
	(I) IV infusion (unlicensed) via syringe pump for variceal bleeds.	Dilute dose to 10ml with N/S i.e. to a ratio of not less than 1:1 and not more than 1:9 by volume.	10 to 20 hours.	To reduce local discomfort, let solution reach room temperature before injection. When administered subcutaneously, smaller volumes cause less discomfort. Diluted solutions should be discarded after 24 hours (local practice).	

DRUG AND FORMULATION	METHOD	INSTRUCTION FOR DILUTION AND SUITABLE DILUENT	ADMINISTER OVER	COMMENTS	COMPATIBILITY
Omeprazole (unlicensed) Vial 40mg containing 42.6mg of the lyophilised sodium salt	(I) IV infusion.	Reconstitute vial with sufficient (~10ml) N/S or G from a 100ml bag. Then inject reconstituted solution from the vial into the same 100ml bag.	20-30 minutes.	**Acute Events Which May Accompany Administration** Bradycardia, tachycardia, hypertension, monitor blood pressure and heart rate. Extravasation may cause tissue damage; for management guidelines see section A 7. **pH:** 9-10 **Flush:** N/S. **Sodium content:** negligible. **Other comments** Revert to oral therapy as soon as possible. Use infusion in N/S within 12 hours, or 6 hours if in G.	**Incompatible:** Do not infuse with other drugs or infusion fluids.
Ondansetron Ampoule 4mg/2ml, 8mg/4ml	IV bolus.	May be diluted with N/S or G.	2-5 minutes.	**Acute Events Which May Accompany Administration** Extravasation may cause tissue damage; for management guidelines see section A 7. **pH:** 3.4-3.8 **Flush:** N/S. **Sodium content:** negligible.	**Y-site compatible (but see section A 2.6):** concentration dependent see data sheet. Bleomycin, cisplatin, cyclophosphamide, cytarabine, doxorubicin, etoposide, fluorouracil, ifosfamide, mannitol 10%, methotrexate, potassium chloride. **Incompatible:** aciclovir, amphotericin, amsacrine, alkaline agents.
	IM. (maximum volume at one site 2ml).	Ready diluted.			
	(C) S/C infusion (local practice).	Dilute to a suitable volume with W or N/S.			

Notes

a) For abbreviations used in the table see section A 2.4

b) Prepare a fresh infusion every 24 hours unless otherwise specified.

130

DRUG AND FORMULATION	METHOD	INSTRUCTION FOR DILUTION AND SUITABLE DILUENT	ADMINISTER OVER	COMMENTS	COMPATIBILITY
Oxytocin Ampoule 5 units/1ml, 10 units/1ml	(C) IV infusion. via volumetric infusion pump.	**Induction/enhancement of labour:** Dilute 10units/500ml H (local practice).	Consult specialist information	**Acute Events Which May Accompany Administration** Uterine spasm, uterine hyperstimulation, nausea, vomiting and arrhythmias. Monitor maternal and foetal heart rate and blood pressure. Rapid infusion may cause an acute short lasting hypotension accompanied by flushing and reflex tachycardia. Extravasation may cause tissue damage; for management guidelines see section A 7.	**Compatible fluids:** N/S, G, Ringers solution. **Y-site compatible (but see section A 2.6):** Hep/S, potassium chloride. **Incompatible:** solutions containing sodium metabisulphite.
		Incomplete, inevitable or missed abortion: 5 units by slow IV bolus followed by infusion of 40 units/500ml H if necessary.	20-40 milliunits/min or higher.	**pH:** 3.7-4.3 **Flush:** N/S.	
		Treatment of postpartum uterine haemorrhage (PPH): 5 units by slow IV bolus followed by an infusion of 5-20units in 500ml H if necessary.	Dependent upon patient.	**Other comments** When high doses are administered over long periods, an electrolyte containing diluent (not glucose) must be used. The volume of infused fluid should be kept low and fluid intake by mouth restricted, to prevent water intoxication and associated hyponatraemia.	
	IV bolus.	**Prevention of PPH:** 5 units, ready diluted.	2-3 minutes.		
	IM (unlicensed).	**PPH prophylaxis:** ready diluted.			

DRUG AND FORMULATION	METHOD	INSTRUCTION FOR DILUTION AND SUITABLE DILUENT	ADMINISTER OVER	COMMENTS	COMPATIBILITY
Pabrinex IVHP Ampoule No. 1 contains pyridoxine 50mg, riboflavine 4mg, thiamine 250mg in 5ml Ampoule No. 2 contains ascorbic acid 500mg, glucose 1g, nicotinamide 160mg in 5ml	(I) IV infusion (preferred method).	Draw the contents of ampoule No. 1 and 2 (one pair of ampoules) into one syringe and mix. Add to 50-100ml N/S.	15-30 minutes.	**Acute Events Which May Accompany Administration** Anaphylaxis. Mild allergic reactions such as sneezing or mild asthma are warning signs that further injections may give rise to anaphylactic shock. **pH:** 4.6 **Flush:** N/S. **Other comments** In thiamine deficiency avoid parenteral glucose as it may worsen symptoms and increase thiamine requirements.	
	IV bolus.	Draw the contents of each pair of ampoules into one syringe and mix.	10 minutes.		
Pamidronate Vial 15mg, 30mg	(I) IV infusion preferably into a large vein.	Reconstitute each 15mg with 5ml of W. Further dilute with N/S, G or G/S. The final concentration should not exceed 60mg/250ml.	Maximum rate 60mg/hour. However in renal impairment the recommended rate is 20mg/hour.	**Acute Events Which May Accompany Administration** Hyper or hypotension, monitor blood pressure. Fever and flu-like symptoms, treat with paracetamol. Local reactions such as pain, redness, induration, phlebitis and thrombophlebitis. **pH:** 6-7.4 **Flush:** N/S. **Sodium content:** negligible.	**Incompatible:** calcium containing solutions.

Notes

a) For abbreviations used in the table see section A 2.4

b) Prepare a fresh infusion every 24 hours unless otherwise specified.

DRUG AND FORMULATION	METHOD	INSTRUCTION FOR DILUTION AND SUITABLE DILUENT	ADMINISTER OVER	COMMENTS	COMPATIBILITY
Pancreozymin	See cholecystokinin (CCK)				
Pancuronium Ampoule 4mg/2ml	IV bolus.	May be diluted with G or N/S. Neonates: dilute with pancuronium diluent (unlicensed).	30 seconds.	**Acute Events Which May Accompany Administration** Tachycardia and rise in arterial pressure and cardiac output. Monitor heart rate and blood pressure. Extravasation may cause tissue damage; for management guidelines see section A 7. **pH:** 3.8-4.2	**Y-site compatible (but see section A 2.6):** alfentanil, aminophylline, chlormethiazole, co-trimoxazole, dobutamine, fentanyl, gentamicin, heparin, hydrocortisone sodium succinate, isoprenaline, midazolam, morphine, propofol, sodium nitroprusside. **Incompatible:** phenobarbitone.
	(I) or (C) IV infusion via a syringe pump (unlicensed).	May be diluted with G or N/S.	Dependent on patient response.	**Flush:** N/S or G. **Sodium content:** 0.28mmol/2ml.	
	IM (unlicensed).	Ready diluted.			
Papaveretum Ampoule 15.4mg/1ml	IM or S/C (preferred method) see 'Other comments'.	Ready diluted.		**Acute Events Which May Accompany Administration** Respiratory depression, hypotension, sedation, anaphylaxis, nausea and vomiting. Monitor blood pressure, heart rate, respiratory rate, sedation score.	
	(C) IV infusion via syringe pump (unlicensed).	Dilute with N/S or G.		**pH:** 2.5-4 **Flush:** N/S. **Sodium content:** negligible. **Other comments**	
	IV bolus.	Dilute with W, N/S or G.	2-3 minutes.	IM injection is preferred to S/C as it is less irritant. IM injections should be injected into large muscle mass to	

DRUG AND FORMULATION	METHOD	INSTRUCTION FOR DILUTION AND SUITABLE DILUENT	ADMINISTER OVER	COMMENTS	COMPATIBILITY
				avoid nerve trunks.	
Pentamidine Vial 300mg	(I) IV infusion with patient supine.	Reconstitute with 3-5ml W. Withdraw the appropriate dose and dilute with 250ml N/S or G.	Minimum 1 hour. For prehydration see 'Other comments'.	**Acute Events Which May Accompany** **Administration** May cause sudden, severe hypotension; to reduce risk - keep patient supine. Baseline blood pressure should be established prior to infusion and monitored every 15 minutes during and one hour post infusion. **pH:** 4.5-6.5 (5% solution) **Flush:** N/S or G. **Sodium content:** nil. **Displacement:** 0.15ml/300mg. Add 4.85ml W to 300mg vial to give a concentration of 60mg/1ml.	Do not infuse with other drugs.
	IM (not recommended in HIV).	Reconstitute with 3ml W.		**Other comments** Consider pre-hydration to reduce renal toxicity with 500ml-1 litre N/S, depending on fluid tolerance.	

Notes

a) For abbreviations used in the table see section A 2.4

b) Prepare a fresh infusion every 24 hours unless otherwise specified.

DRUG AND FORMULATION	METHOD	INSTRUCTION FOR DILUTION AND SUITABLE DILUENT	ADMINISTER OVER	COMMENTS	COMPATIBILITY
Pethidine Ampoule 50mg/1ml, 100mg/2ml	IV bolus.	May be diluted with W, N/S or G to a concentration of 10mg/1ml.	2-3 minutes.	<u>**Acute Events Which May Accompany Administration**</u> Respiratory depression, hypotension, sedation, anaphylaxis, nausea and vomiting. Monitor blood pressure, heart rate, respiratory rate, sedation score.	May be mixed in an infusion with amphotericin (local practice). <u>**Y-site compatible (but see section A 2.6)**</u>:
	(C) IV infusion (unlicensed) via volumetric infusion or syringe pump.	Dilute with N/S, G or H.		<u>**pH:**</u> 4.5-6 <u>**Flush:**</u> N/S or G. <u>**Sodium content:**</u> nil. <u>**Other comments**</u>	amphotericin, bumetanide, hyoscine butylbromide, glycopyrronium, insulin, labetalol, potassium chloride, propranolol.
	IM into large muscle mass. See 'Other comments'.	Ready diluted.		The IM route is preferred to S/C for repeated injections. This is because of occurrence of irritation and induration at the S/C injection site.	<u>**Incompatible:**</u> aciclovir, aminophylline, heparin, imipenem, ketorolac, phenobarbitone, phenytoin.
	S/C. See 'Other comments'.	Ready diluted.			

DRUG AND FORMULATION	METHOD	INSTRUCTION FOR DILUTION AND SUITABLE DILUENT	ADMINISTER OVER	COMMENTS	COMPATIBILITY
Phenobarbitone Ampoule 15mg/1ml, 30mg/1ml, 60mg/1ml, 200mg/1ml	IV bolus.	Dilute to 10 times its own volume with W immediately before use.	**Adults/ neonates:** Maximum rate 1mg/kg/min not exceeding 60mg/minute.	**Acute Events Which May Accompany Administration** Sedation, hypotension, tachycardia, respiratory depression. Monitor sedation score, respiratory rate, heart rate and blood pressure. Extravasation may cause tissue damage; for management guidelines see section A 7.	**Incompatible:** acidic solutions including, chlorpromazine, droperidol, ephedrine, ketamine, pancuronium, pethidine, vancomycin.
	(I) IV infusion via syringe pump.	As above.		**pH:** 9-10.5 **Flush:** N/S.	
	IM.	May dilute with W to a suitable volume.		**Sodium content per ampoule:** negligible.	
Phenoxy-benzamine Ampoule 100mg/2ml	(I) IV infusion via volumetric infusion pump. Infuse into a large vein.	Dilute with 200-500ml N/S.	Minimum 2 hours (give 1/3rd of dose over first hour).	**Acute Events Which May Accompany Administration** Hypotension, monitor blood pressure. Extravasation may cause tissue damage; for management guidelines see section A 7. **pH:** 2.5-3.1 **Flush:** N/S. **Other comments** Discard infusion 4 hours after dilution.	

Notes

a) For abbreviations used in the table see section A 2.4

b) Prepare a fresh infusion every 24 hours unless otherwise specified.

DRUG AND FORMULATION	METHOD	INSTRUCTION FOR DILUTION AND SUITABLE DILUENT	ADMINISTER OVER	COMMENTS	COMPATIBILITY
Phentolamine mesylate Ampoule 10mg/1ml	IV bolus.	Ready diluted.	Rapidly.	**Acute Events Which May Accompany Administration** Tachycardia and arrhythmias and hypotension, monitor **ECG** and blood pressure. **Flush:** N/S, G or G/S.	
	IM.	Ready diluted.		**pH:** 5	
Phenylephrine Ampoule 10mg/1ml (10,000micrograms/ 1ml)	IV bolus.	Dilute 1mg (1,000micrograms) with 1ml W.	100-500micrograms over 3-5 minutes.	**Acute Events Which May Accompany Administration** Respiratory distress, hypertension, headache, tremor, bradycardia, palpitations and vomiting. Can cause severe peripheral and visceral vasoconstriction and volume depletion.	**Y-site compatible (but see section A 2.6):** aminophylline, amiodarone, dobutamine, heparin, lignocaine. **Incompatible:** phenytoin.
	(I) IV infusion via volumetric infusion pump.	Add 5-20mg (5,000-20,000 micrograms) to 500ml of N/S or G.	Up to 180micro-grams/minute reduced according to response to 30-60micrograms/ minute.	Extravasation may cause local tissue necrosis, for management guidelines see section A 7. Monitor blood pressure and heart rate during IV infusions and regularly post IM or S/C injections. Ensure patient is not volume depleted prior to infusion. **pH:** 4.5-6.5 **Flush:** N/S or G.	
	IM or S/C.	Ready diluted.	Maximum dose 5mg.		

DRUG AND FORMULATION	METHOD	INSTRUCTION FOR DILUTION AND SUITABLE DILUENT	ADMINISTER OVER	COMMENTS	COMPATIBILITY
Phenytoin sodium Ampoule 250mg/5ml	IV bolus (preferred method). Inject via a large needle into a large vein.	Unless essential do not dilute as precipitation may occur.	**Adults:** Maximum rate 50mg/minute. **Neonates:** 1-3mg/kg/minute.	**Acute Events Which May Accompany Administration** Arrhythmias, **ECG** monitoring recommended. Hypotension monitor blood pressure. Respiratory depression. Extravasation may cause tissue damage; for management guidelines see section A 7.	**Y-site compatible (but see section A 2.6):** chlormethiazole. **Incompatible:** ciprofloxacin, clindamycin, insulin, lignocaine, morphine, pethidine, phenylephrine, procainamide.
	(I) IV infusion via a syringe or volumetric infusion pump. Inject via a large needle into a large vein.	Dilute in 50-100ml N/S to a final concentration not exceeding 10mg/1ml. Stable for 1 hour. Use an in-line 0.2-0.50 micron filter. Do not use if solution is hazy or contains precipitate.		**pH:** 12 **Flush:** N/S. **Sodium content:** 0.91mmol/250mg. **Other comments** Plasma level monitoring is required.	
Phosphates neutral Polyfusor 50mmol/500ml	(I) IV infusion.	Ready diluted.	Usual maximum rate 9mmol of phosphate over 12 hours (7.5ml/hour). Faster rates are used on ITU i.e. 50mmol/24 hours (local practice).	**Acute Events Which May Accompany Administration** Oedema and hypotension, monitor blood pressure. Doses exceeding 9mmol/12 hours may cause hypocalcaemia and metastatic calcification, monitor calcium, phosphate, potassium, other electrolytes and renal function. **pH:** 7-7.8 **Flush:** N/S.	

Notes

a) For abbreviations used in the table see section A 2.4

b) Prepare a fresh infusion every 24 hours unless otherwise specified.

DRUG AND FORMULATION	METHOD	INSTRUCTION FOR DILUTION AND SUITABLE DILUENT	ADMINISTER OVER	COMMENTS	COMPATIBILITY
Phytomenadione (Konakion MM) - new formulation	IV bolus.	Ready diluted.	2-3 minutes.	**Acute Events Which May Accompany Administration** Possible anaphylactoid reactions. **pH:** 5.5-6.3 (Konakion MM), 5-7.5 (Konakion) **Flush:** G.	
Ampoule 10mg/1ml	(I) IV infusion.	Add to 100ml G before administration.	15-30 minutes.	**Other comments** Konakion 1mg/0.5ml should be used in infants.	
Phytomenadione (Konakion)	IM.	Ready diluted.			
Ampoule 1mg/0.5ml	IV bolus.	Ready diluted.	Maximum rate 1mg/minute.		
Piperacillin and tazobactam Vial 2.25g containing piperacillin 2g, tazobactam 250mg.	IV bolus.	Reconstitute the 2.25g vial with 10ml of W or N/S, and the 4.5g vial with 20ml of W or N/S.	3-5 minutes.	**Acute Events Which May Accompany Administration** Thrombophlebitis. Anaphylaxis. **pH:** 5-7 **Flush:** N/S. **Sodium content:** 4.5mmol/2.25g, 9mmol/4.5g.	**Y-site compatible (but see section A 2.6):** folinic acid, potassium chloride. **Incompatible:** amphotericin.
Vial 4.5g containing piperacillin 4g, tazobactam 500mg.	(I) IV infusion.	Reconstitute as above then dilute to a convenient volume with N/S, G or G/S.	20-30 minutes.	**Displacement:** 1.6ml/2.25g Add 8.4ml diluent to 2.25g vial to give a concentration of 225mg/1ml.	

DRUG AND FORMULATION	METHOD	INSTRUCTION FOR DILUTION AND SUITABLE DILUENT	ADMINISTER OVER	COMMENTS	COMPATIBILITY
Potassium canrenoate Ampoule 200mg/10ml	IV bolus preferably not into small vein.	Ready diluted.	Maximum rate 100mg/minute.	**Acute Events Which May Accompany Administration** If the undiluted solution is injected too quickly pain and irritation at the injection site may occur. Transient confusion may occur during high dose therapy ($\geq$ 1g daily). Extravasation may cause tissue damage; for management guidelines see section A 7.	Do not infuse with other drugs.
	(I) IV infusion.	Dilute to 250ml with N/S or G (G is preferred if ascites present).	90 minutes.	**pH:** 10.7-11.2 **Flush:** N/S or G. **Other comments** Use infusion within 12 hours.	

Notes

a) For abbreviations used in the table see section A 2.4

b) Prepare a fresh infusion every 24 hours unless otherwise specified.

DRUG AND FORMULATION	METHOD	INSTRUCTION FOR DILUTION AND SUITABLE DILUENT	ADMINISTER OVER	COMMENTS	COMPATIBILITY
Potassium chloride Infusion bag 10mmol in 500ml N/S, 20mmol in 500ml N/S, 20mmol in 1 litre N/S, 40mmol in 1 litre N/S, 10mmol in 500ml G, 20mmol in 1 litre G, 20mmol in 500ml G, 40mmol in 1 litre G, 10mmol in 500ml	(C) IV infusion into a peripheral line via a volumetric infusion pump.	Maximum concentration 40mmol/litre. Use ready prepared infusion bags containing potassium 20mmol/litre and 40mmol/litre in N/S, G or G/S.	**Adults:** Usual suggested maximum rate 20mmol potassium/hour. **Children:** Usual maximum rate 0.5mmol potassium/kg/hour.	**Acute Events Which May Accompany Administration** ECG monitoring should be used when the rate exceeds 20mmol/hour. Administration of concentrations exceeding 40mmol over a period of less than 1 hour poses a serious risk of asystole. Pain or phlebitis may occur during peripheral administration of solutions containing more than 30mmol/litre of potassium. Extravasation may cause tissue damage; for management guidelines see section A 7. **pH:** 4-8 **Flush:** N/S.	**Y-site compatible (but see section A 2.6):** aciclovir, adrenaline, amiodarone, aminophylline, atracurium, atropine, calcium gluconate, ceftazidime, chlormethiazole, ciprofloxacin, clindamycin, digoxin, dobutamine, dopamine, doxapram, fentanyl, flucloxacillin, fluconazole, frusemide, heparin, human albumin 4.5%, hydralazine, hydrocortisone sodium succinate, insulin, isoprenaline, labetalol, lignocaine, magnesium sulphate, mannitol, mesna, methyldopa, metronidazole, morphine, neostigmine, noradrenaline, ondansetron, oxytocin, pethidine, piperacillin/tazobactam, procainamide, propranolol, ranitidine, sodium bicarbonate, suxamethonium, trimetaphan. **Incompatible:** amphotericin, methylprednisolone sodium succinate.
	(C) or (I) IV infusion into a central line via a syringe or volumetric infusion pump.	Dilute to required concentration with N/S, G or G/S and MIX THOROUGHLY. Concentrations greater than 40mmol/litre are only given in UCLH on ITU, Coronary Care Unit, Neonatal Unit, Haematology and Oncology wards.			
Potassium G/S, 20mmol in 1 litre G/S, 20mmol in 500ml G/S, 40mmol in 1 litre G/S Ampoule 1.5g/10ml (20 mmol)	(I) or (C) IV infusion via a	Dilute with N/S, G or G/S to a usual maximum concentration	**Adults:** Usual maximum rate	**Acute Events Which May Accompany Administration**	**Incompatible:** calcium salts.

DRUG AND FORMULATION	METHOD	INSTRUCTION FOR DILUTION AND SUITABLE DILUENT	ADMINISTER OVER	COMMENTS	COMPATIBILITY
phosphate (unlicensed) Ampoule 17.42%, 5ml containing potassium 10mmol/5ml and phosphate 5mmol/5ml	syringe or volumetric infusion pump.	of 40mmol potassium/litre. **Children:** dilute 3ml with at least 60ml N/S, G or G/S for peripheral and 25ml for central administration.	9mmol of phosphate over 12 hours. Faster rates are used on ITU. **Children:** seek expert advice.	**ECG** should be monitored when the rate exceeds 20mmol/hour of potassium. Administration of concentrations exceeding 40mmol of potassium over a period of less than 1 hour poses a serious risk of asystole. Pain or phlebitis may occur during peripheral administration of solutions containing more than 30mmol/litre of potassium. Oedema and hypotension, monitor blood pressure. Doses of phosphate exceeding 9mmol/12 hours may cause hypocalcaemia and metastatic calcification, monitor calcium, phosphate, potassium, other electrolytes and renal function. Extravasation may cause tissue damage; for management guidelines see section A 7. **Flush:** N/S.	

Notes

a) For abbreviations used in the table see section A 2.4

b) Prepare a fresh infusion every 24 hours unless otherwise specified.

DRUG AND FORMULATION	METHOD	INSTRUCTION FOR DILUTION AND SUITABLE DILUENT	ADMINISTER OVER	COMMENTS	COMPATIBILITY
Procainamide Vial 1g/10ml	IV bolus (for acute control of tachy-arrhythmia).	May be diluted with G.	Maximum rate 50mg/minute.	**Acute Events Which May Accompany Administration** Hypotension and myocardial toxicity, monitor blood pressure and **ECG**. Hypersensitivity reactions. **pH:** 4.5-5.5 **Flush:** G or N/S.	**Y-site compatible (but see section A 2.6):** amiodarone, dobutamine, heparin, lignocaine, potassium chloride. **Incompatible:** phenytoin.
	(I) and then (C) IV infusion via volumetric infusion pump (for suppression of chronic arrhythmias).	Dilute to 2-4mg/1ml with G.	Loading dose: infuse 500mg-600mg over 25-30 minutes then infuse maintenance dose at 2-6mg/minute.		
Prochlorperazine Ampoule 12.5mg/1ml	IV bolus (unlicensed).	Dilute 1 part with 9 parts W by volume before administration.	Maximum rate 1.25mg/minute.	**Acute Events Which May Accompany Administration** Venospasm and postural hypotension, monitor blood pressure and heart rate. Rapid administration may irritate veins. Extravasation may cause tissue damage; for management guidelines see section A 7. **pH:** 3.9-4.5 **Flush:** N/S.	Do not infuse with other drugs.
	Deep IM.	Ready diluted.		**Sodium content:** negligible.	
Procyclidine	IV bolus.	Ready diluted.	Rapidly.	**pH:** 3.9-4.5 **Flush:** N/S.	
Ampoule 10mg/2ml	IM.	Ready diluted.			
Promethazine	Deep IM	Ready diluted.		**Acute Events Which May Accompany**	**Y-site compatible (but see**

DRUG AND FORMULATION	METHOD	INSTRUCTION FOR DILUTION AND SUITABLE DILUENT	ADMINISTER OVER	COMMENTS	COMPATIBILITY
Ampoule 25mg/1ml	(preferred method).			**Administration** Pain at injection site. Hypotension, monitor blood pressure. Extravasation may cause tissue damage; for management guidelines see section A 7.	**section A 2.6):** G, N/S, buprenorphine. **Incompatible:** alkaline agents, ketorolac.
	IV bolus.	Dilute 1 part with 9 parts W before administration.	Give slowly. Maximum rate 25mg/minute.	**pH:** 5-6 **Flush:** N/S.	
Propofol Ampoule 200mg/20ml Vial 500mg/50ml, 1000mg/100ml	IV bolus.	Ready diluted. May be administered into a Y-site (close to the injection site) of infusions of N/S, G or G/S.	**Adults:** 2-2.5mg/kg at rate of 20-40mg every 10 seconds.	**Acute Events Which May Accompany Administration** Hypotension, monitor airways obstruction and oxygen desaturation. **pH:** 7-7.1	**Y-site compatible (but see section A 2.6):** alfentanil, atropine, fentanyl, morphine (local practice), pancuronium, suxamethonium. **Incompatible:** atracurium.
	(C) IV infusion via syringe or volumetric infusion pump.	Infuse undiluted or dilute with G to a concentration between 2-10mg/1ml.	Dependent on indication, see package insert.	**Flush:** N/S. **Other comments** Discard any unused diluted infusion after 6 hours.	
Propranolol Ampoule 1mg/1ml	IV bolus.	May be diluted with N/S or G.	**Adults and children:** Maximum rate 1mg/minute.	**Acute Events Which May Accompany Administration** Bradycardia, monitor ECG. Extravasation may cause tissue damage; for management guidelines see section A 7. **pH:** 3 **Flush:** N/S. **Sodium content:** nil.	**Y-site compatible (but see section A 2.6):** heparin, morphine, pethidine, potassium chloride. **Incompatible:** decomposes rapidly at alkaline pH.

Notes
a) For abbreviations used in the table see section A 2.4
b) Prepare a fresh infusion every 24 hours unless otherwise specified.

144

DRUG AND FORMULATION	METHOD	INSTRUCTION FOR DILUTION AND SUITABLE DILUENT	ADMINISTER OVER	COMMENTS	COMPATIBILITY
Prostacyclin	See epoprostenol				
Prostaglandin E1	See alprostadil				
Protamine sulphate Ampoule 50mg/5ml, 100mg/10ml	IV bolus via a peripheral vein.	May be diluted with N/S or G.	10 minutes.	**Acute Events Which May Accompany Administration** Monitor APTT coagulation tests. Rapid administration may cause hypotension, bradycardia and dyspnoea. Extravasation may cause tissue damage; for management guidelines see section A 7. **pH:** 2.5-3.5 **Flush:** N/S. **Sodium content:** 0.75mmol/5ml.	
Protirelin Ampoule 200mg/2ml	IV bolus (diagnostic test).	Ready diluted.	30 seconds.	**Acute Events Which May Accompany Administration** Hyper or hypotension, tachycardia and bronchospasm. The patient should be lying down during administration to reduce hypotension. Monitor blood pressure and heart rate. **pH:** 4.5-6.5 **Flush:** N/S.	
Pyridoxine (unlicensed) Ampoule 100mg/2ml	IV bolus.	Dilute with N/S.	Minimum 5 minutes.	**Acute Events Which May Accompany Administration** Hypersensitivity reactions. **Flush:** N/S.	
Quinine	(I) IV infusion via volumetric	Add required dose to 250ml preferably in N/S (otherwise	4 hours.	**Acute Events Which May Accompany Administration**	

DRUG AND FORMULATION	METHOD	INSTRUCTION FOR DILUTION AND SUITABLE DILUENT	ADMINISTER OVER	COMMENTS	COMPATIBILITY
dihydrochloride Ampoule 300mg/1ml, 600mg/2ml	infusion pump.	G or G10%). Normal maximum concentration is 2.4mg/1ml (local practice).		Hypoglycaemia, monitor blood glucose levels. Cinchonism including tinnitis, headache, nausea, abdominal pain and visual disturbances. Fever and hypersensitivity such as flushing of skin and intense pruritis. Extravasation may cause tissue damage; for management guidelines see section A 7.	
	IM into anterior thigh.	Dilute in N/S to 60mg/1ml and give half dose into each thigh (local practice).		**pH:** 2-3 **Flush:** N/S or G.	
Ranitidine Ampoule 50mg/2ml	IV bolus.	Dilute each 50mg with a minimum of 20ml N/S or G.	Minimum 2 minutes.	**Acute Events Which May Accompany Administration** Rapid administration may occasionally produce bradycardia. **pH:** 6.7-7.3	**Y-site compatible (but see section A 2.6):** amikacin, aminophylline, flucloxacillin, frusemide, glyceryl trinitrate, heparin, labetalol, potassium chloride, sodium bicarbonate.
	(I) IV infusion.	Dilute to 100ml with N/S or G.	25mg/hour for 2 hours.	**Flush:** N/S, G or G/S. **Sodium content:** negligible.	**Incompatible:** amphotericin, diazepam, midazolam, methotrimeprazine.
	(C) IV infusion following initial IV bolus.		125-250 micrograms/kg/hour.		
	Deep IM.	Ready diluted.			

Notes

a) For abbreviations used in the table see section A 2.4

b) Prepare a fresh infusion every 24 hours unless otherwise specified.

DRUG AND FORMULATION	METHOD	INSTRUCTION FOR DILUTION AND SUITABLE DILUENT	ADMINISTER OVER	COMMENTS	COMPATIBILITY
Rifampicin Vial 300mg, 600mg	(I) IV infusion.	Reconstitute with diluent provided and shake vigorously for 30-60 seconds then dilute to a maximum concentration of 600mg in 500ml N/S or G.	2-3 hours.	**Acute Events Which May Accompany Administration** May colour the urine, sputum and tears orange-red. Soft contact lens may be permanently discoloured and should not be inserted during therapy. **pH:** 8-8.8	Do not infuse with other drugs.
	(I) IV infusion for fluid restriction (unlicensed).	Reconstitute with diluent provided then dilute "Rifadin" brand 300-600mg in 100ml preferably with G, otherwise N/S. The maximum dilution of the "Rimactane" brand is 300mg in 100ml G or N/S.	30 minutes for "Rifadin". 2-3 hours for "Rimactane".	**Flush:** N/S. **Sodium content:** less than 0.5mmol/600mg. **Displacement:** 0.24ml/300mg vial. Add 4.76ml diluent to 300mg vial to give a concentration of 60mg/1ml. **Other comments** Discard infusion after 4 hours.	
Ritodrine Ampoule 50mg/5ml	(C) IV infusion via syringe pump (preferred method).	Dilute to 3,000micrograms/1ml with G i.e. 150mg added to 35ml of G to give a total volume of 50ml.	Variable, see package insert. Maximum rate 350micrograms/minute.	**Acute Events Which May Accompany Administration** Pulmonary oedema, monitor fluid balance. Monitor maternal heart rate as it may increase leading to palpitations. Closely monitor blood glucose levels in diabetic patients. **pH:** 4.8-5.5 **Flush:** G or N/S. **Other comments**	
	(C) IV infusion without a syringe pump.	Dilute to 300micrograms/1ml with G i.e. 150mg in 500ml of G.			
	IM.	Ready diluted.		The diluent should usually be G, but N/S can be used if clinically indicated e.g. diabetes. The volume of infusion fluid should be kept to a minimum.	
Rocuronium	IV bolus.	Ready diluted.	15-30 seconds.	**Acute Events Which May Accompany**	

DRUG AND FORMULATION	METHOD	INSTRUCTION FOR DILUTION AND SUITABLE DILUENT	ADMINISTER OVER	COMMENTS	COMPATIBILITY
Ampoule 50mg/5ml, 100mg/10ml				**Administration** High doses (greater than 0.9mg/kg) may cause an increase in heart rate.	
	(C) IV infusion.	May be diluted with N/S, G or G/S.	0.3-0.6mg/kg/hour. Adjust to response.	**pH:** 3.5-4 **Flush:** G or N/S. **Sodium content:** 1.5mmol/50mg.	
Salbutamol	IV bolus.	Dilute 500micrograms/1ml ampoule to 50micrograms/1ml with W.	3-5 minutes.	**Acute Events Which May Accompany Administration**	
Ampoule 500micrograms/1ml 5mg/5ml for infusion	(C) IV infusion for asthma.	Dilute to 10micrograms/1ml with G (i.e. 5ml of 5mg/5ml added to 495ml of G).		Increases in heart rate, monitor **ECG**. Rarely hypersensitivity reactions including urticaria, bronchospasm and hypotension, monitor blood pressure.	
	(C) IV infusion for premature labour via syringe pump.	Dilute to 200micrograms/1ml with G (i.e. 10ml of 5mg/5ml added to 40ml of G).		Extravasation may cause tissue damage; for management guidelines see section A 7. **pH:** 3.5 **Flush:** N/S or G.	
	(C) IV infusion for premature labour if syringe pump is unavailable.	Dilute to 20micrograms/1ml with G (i.e. 10ml of 5mg/5ml added to 490ml of G).		**Sodium content:** 0.15mmol/1ml. **Other comments** Salbutamol may be diluted with W, N/S or G.	
	IM or S/C. See 'Other comments'.	Ready diluted.		IM injection may produce slight pain or stinging.	
Secretin	IV bolus.	Dissolve contents of vial in	1 minute.	**Acute Events Which May Accompany**	

Notes

a) For abbreviations used in the table see section A 2.4

b) Prepare a fresh infusion every 24 hours unless otherwise specified.

DRUG AND FORMULATION	METHOD	INSTRUCTION FOR DILUTION AND SUITABLE DILUENT	ADMINISTER OVER	COMMENTS	COMPATIBILITY
(unlicensed) Vial 75 clinical units (cu)		7.5ml N/S, producing a concentration of 10cu/1ml. Avoid vigorous shaking.	See 'Other comments' for test dose.	**Administration** Allergic reactions since porcine derived. **pH:** 2.5-5 **Flush:** N/S. **Other comments** Give a test dose of 0.1-1cu, wait 1 minute if there is no allergic reaction, administer the recommended dose.	
Sodium benzoate (unlicensed) Ampoule 1g/5ml, 5g/25ml	(I) or (C) IV infusion.	Seek specialist advice.		**Acute Events Which May Accompany Administration** Vomiting. **Sodium content:** 3.5mmol/500mg.	
Sodium bicarbonate Infusion bag 1.26%	(C) IV infusion.	Use ready prepared infusions when possible. May be diluted with N/S or G.	Variable.	**Acute Events Which May Accompany Administration** Extravasation may cause tissue damage; for management guidelines see section A 7. **pH:** 7-8.5	**Y-site compatible (but see section A 2.6):** amphotericin, chlormethiazole. fentanyl, fluconazole. methotrexate, potassium chloride, ranitidine.

149

DRUG AND FORMULATION	METHOD	INSTRUCTION FOR DILUTION AND SUITABLE DILUENT	ADMINISTER OVER	COMMENTS	COMPATIBILITY
500ml Polyfusor 4.2% 500ml				**Flush:** N/S or G.	
Infusion bottle 8.4% 100ml	IV bolus.	Ready diluted.		**Other comments** Concentrations over 1.26% should be given via a central line.	**Incompatible:** ceftazidime, cefuroxime, cisplatin, dobutamine, dopamine, doxapram, insulin, isoprenaline, labetalol, morphine,
Ampoule 4.2% 10ml, 8.4% 10ml	(I) IV infusion.	Use ready prepared infusions when possible. May be diluted with N/S or G.	Variable.		noradrenaline, solutions containing calcium, magnesium or phosphate.
Sodium calciumedetate Ampoule 1000mg/5ml	(I) IV infusion via volumetric infusion pump. IM. See 'Other comments'. S/C.	Dilute with 250-500ml N/S or G [maximum concentration 3% (3000mg/100ml)]. Ready diluted.	Minimum 1 hour.	**Acute Events Which May Accompany Administration** Thrombophlebitis. **pH:** 6.5-8 **Flush:** N/S. **Sodium content:** 5.3mmol/1000mg. **Other comments** IM injection is painful, add a local anaesthetic.	Do not infuse with other drugs.
Sodium chloride Ampoule 0.9% 2ml, 5ml, 10ml.	(C) or (I) IV infusion.	Use ready prepared infusions when possible.		**Acute Events Which May Accompany Administration** Vein irritation with concentrated solutions. **pH:** 4.5-7	Check under individual drug.

Notes

a) For abbreviations used in the table see section A 2.4

b) Prepare a fresh infusion every 24 hours unless otherwise specified.

DRUG AND FORMULATION	METHOD	INSTRUCTION FOR DILUTION AND SUITABLE DILUENT	ADMINISTER OVER	COMMENTS	COMPATIBILITY
30%, 10ml				**Sodium content:** of 0.9% injection is 150mmol/1 litre. **Other comments** Concentrations over 1.8% should be given via a central line.	
Infusion bags 0.9% 100ml, 250ml, 500ml, 1000ml. 0.45%, 1.8%, 2.7%, 5% 500ml	IV bolus.	Concentrated solutions may be diluted with N/S, G, G/S or H.			
Sodium fusidate Vial 500mg	(I) IV infusion into a central venous line (preferred method).	Reconstitute with 10ml buffered diluent provided then dilute with at least 500ml N/S, G or G/S. **Paediatric information:** Dilute 0.6-0.7ml/kg of buffered drug at least 10 fold with N/S.	2 hours.	**Acute Events Which May Accompany Administration** Pain at injection site. Rapid infusion may cause venospasm, haemolysis of erythrocytes and thrombophlebitis. **pH:** 7.4-7.6 after reconstitution with buffer. **Flush:** N/S. **Sodium and phosphate content:** When reconstituted with 10ml buffer contains 3.1mmol sodium and 1.1mmol phosphate. **Displacement:** negligible. **Other comments** G or G/S can be used as diluent but opalescence may occur with more acidic samples. Infusion must be discarded if this occurs.	**Incompatible:** G infusions of 20% and above. Precipitation may occur with solutions of pH less than 7.4.
	(I) IV infusion into large peripheral vein.	As above.	Minimum 6 hours.		
Sodium iodide (unlicensed)	IV bolus.	May dilute with N/S.	3-5 minutes.	**Flush:** N/S.	
Ampoule	(I) IV infusion.	Dilute dose with N/S 1 litre.	8-24 hours		

DRUG AND FORMULATION	METHOD	INSTRUCTION FOR DILUTION AND SUITABLE DILUENT	ADMINISTER OVER	COMMENTS	COMPATIBILITY
100mg/5ml			(or obtain expert opinion).		
Sodium nitroprusside Vial 50mg	(C) IV infusion via syringe or volumetric infusion pump.	ITU local practice: Reconstitute vial with 2ml G provided then further dilute to 50mg/50ml in G or N/S. Alternatively reconstitute vial with 2ml G provided then further dilute in 250 - 1,000ml G or N/S (maximum concentration of 200micrograms/1ml).	Increase rate slowly until desired effect occurs. Discontinue infusion gradually over 10-30 minutes.	**Acute Events Which May Accompany Administration** Hypotension, monitor blood pressure. Rapid reduction in blood pressure can lead to nausea, vomiting, headache and abdominal pain. These effects can be reduced by slowing infusion rate. Extravasation may cause tissue damage; for management guidelines see section A 7. **pH:** 3.5-6 (in G) **Do not flush** - replace giving set. **Sodium content:** 0.34mmol/50mg. **Displacement:** negligible. **Other comments** Protect infusion from light. A faint brown tint in the infusion solution is normal. Do not use if highly coloured. If more than a few days therapy monitor blood thiocyanate levels.	**Y-site compatible (but see section A 2.6):** atracurium, dobutamine, dopamine (both drugs in N/S), glyceryl trinitrate, lignocaine, pancuronium.
Sodium phenylbutyrate (unlicensed)	(I) or (C) IV infusion.	Seek specialist advice.		**Acute Events Which May Accompany Administration** Nausea, vomiting, irritability.	

Notes

a) For abbreviations used in the table see section A 2.4

b) Prepare a fresh infusion every 24 hours unless otherwise specified.

DRUG AND FORMULATION	METHOD	INSTRUCTION FOR DILUTION AND SUITABLE DILUENT	ADMINISTER OVER	COMMENTS	COMPATIBILITY
Vial 1g/5ml				<u>Sodium content:</u> 2.7mmol/500mg.	
Sodium stibogluconate Vial equivalent to 100mg/1ml pentavalent antimony, 100ml	IV bolus.	Ready diluted. Draw up dose through a stainless steel 5 micron filter. Do not administer through filter (local practice).	5 minutes.	**Acute Events Which May Accompany Administration** Rapid administration may cause local thrombosis. If coughing vomiting or substernal pain occur discontinue administration. ECG monitoring is necessary in heart disease.	
	(I) IV infusion (unlicensed).	Draw up dose through a stainless steel 5 micron filter. Dilute dose in 100ml N/S. Do not administer through filter (local practice).	30 minutes.	**pH:** 5.6 **Flush:** W. <u>Other comments</u> The contents of vial can be used for up to 48 hours (local practice). Return to Pharmacy for disposal.	
Sodium valproate Vial 400mg	IV bolus.	Reconstitute with 4ml diluent provided. Due to displacement the resulting concentration is 95mg/1ml. May be diluted with N/S, G or G/S.	3-5 minutes.	**Acute Events Which May Accompany Administration** Vomiting, ataxia, CNS depression - discontinue if these occur. **pH:** 6.8-8.5 **Flush:** N/S, G or G/S.	Do not infuse with other drugs.
	(C) or (I) IV infusion via a syringe or volumetric infusion pump.	As above.		<u>Sodium content:</u> 2.41mmol/400mg vial.	
Sotalol Ampoule 40mg/4ml	IV bolus.	Ready diluted.	Doses up to 60mg over 2-3 minutes. Doses over 60mg minimum 3	**Acute Events Which May Accompany Administration** Bradycardia and hypotension, monitor ECG and blood pressure. **pH:** 4.3-5.2	

153

DRUG AND FORMULATION	METHOD	INSTRUCTION FOR DILUTION AND SUITABLE DILUENT	ADMINISTER OVER	COMMENTS	COMPATIBILITY
Streptokinase Vial 250,000units, 750,000units, 1,500,000units	(C) or (I) IV infusion via volumetric infusion or syringe pump.	Streptase brand: reconstitute all sizes with 5ml N/S. Kabikinase brand: dissolve 250,000unit vial in 5ml W and the 750,000 and 1,500,000 unit vials in 10ml W. Dissolve either brand slowly to avoid foaming. Do not shake. Further dilute to a convenient volume in N/S or G.	Dependent on indication, see package insert for details.	**Flush:** N/S. **Sodium content:** 0.5mmol/ampoule. **Acute Events Which May Accompany Administration** Hypotension and arrhythmias, monitor blood pressure and ECG. Fever, haemorrhage, chills and major allergic reactions. **pH:** 6.8-7.5 **Flush:** N/S. **Displacement:** none. **Other comments** Discard infusion after 12 hours.	**Y-site compatible (but see section A 2.6):** amiodarone, digoxin, flecainide, glyceryl trinitrate, heparin, insulin, lignocaine, magnesium sulphate.
Sulphadiazine Ampoule 1g/4ml	(I) IV infusion (preferred method).	Dilute dose with N/S to a maximum concentration of 50mg/1ml. Preferably dilute required dose in 500ml to 1	Minimum 30-60 minutes.	**Acute Events Which May Accompany Administration** Risk of crystallisation in the urine. A high fluid intake (2.5 to 3.5 litres in 24 hours) should be maintained and	**Incompatible:** acids, iron salts and salts of heavy metals, hydralazine.

Notes

a) For abbreviations used in the table see section A 2.4
b) Prepare a fresh infusion every 24 hours unless otherwise specified.

DRUG AND FORMULATION	METHOD	INSTRUCTION FOR DILUTION AND SUITABLE DILUENT	ADMINISTER OVER	COMMENTS	COMPATIBILITY
		litre of N/S to reduce risk of crystallisation of sulphadiazine in the urine.		urine output should not be less than half that amount. Nausea, give regular anti-emetics half an hour before infusion starts. Extravasation may cause tissue damage; for management guidelines see section A 7. **pH:** 11 (approximately). **Flush:** N/S.	
	Deep IM.	Ready diluted.		**Sodium content:** approximately 4mmol/1g.	
Suxamethonium Ampoule 100mg/2ml	IV bolus.	Ready diluted.	10-30 seconds.	**Acute Events Which May Accompany Administration** Prolonged neuromuscular blockade, bradycardia, hyper and hypotension, muscle pain, anaphylaxis.	**Y-site compatible (but see section A 2.6):** chlormethiazole, heparin, morphine, potassium chloride, propofol. **Incompatible:** Do not mix with anything else in same syringe.
	(C) IV infusion. via volumetric infusion or syringe pump.	Dilute to 1-2mg/1ml with G, N/S or G/S.	2-5mg/minute.	**pH:** 4-4.5 **Flush:** N/S or G. **Sodium content:** negligible.	
	IM.	Ready diluted.			
Teicoplanin Vial 200mg, 400mg	IV bolus.	Add W provided to vial and roll gently until completely reconstituted, taking care to avoid formation of foam. If foam is formed then allow to	3-5 minutes.	**pH:** 7.5 **Flush:** N/S. **Sodium content:** less than 0.5mmol/vial (200mg and 400mg). **Displacement:** 0.59ml/1g. Manufacturer allows for	**Incompatible:** with aminoglycosides.

DRUG AND FORMULATION	METHOD	INSTRUCTION FOR DILUTION AND SUITABLE DILUENT	ADMINISTER OVER	COMMENTS	COMPATIBILITY
		stand for 15 minutes for foam to subside. May be further diluted with N/S, G or G/S.		displacement; when reconstituted as directed 200mg vial contains 200mg/3ml and 400mg vial contains 400mg/3ml.	
	(I) IV infusion.	As above.	30 minutes.		
	IM.	Reconstitute as described for 'IV bolus'.			
Terbutaline	IV bolus.	May be diluted with N/S or G.	Minimum 3-5 minutes.	<u>**Acute Events Which May Accompany Administration**</u>	<u>**Y-site compatible (but see section A 2.6)**</u>: aminophylline, doxapram, insulin.
Ampoule	(C) IV infusion	Dilute 3ml (1.5mg) of the	**Adults:** 1.5-	Tremor, palpitations, dizziness and nervousness.	

Notes

a) For abbreviations used in the table see section A 2.4

b) Prepare a fresh infusion every 24 hours unless otherwise specified.

DRUG AND FORMULATION	METHOD	INSTRUCTION FOR DILUTION AND SUITABLE DILUENT	ADMINISTER OVER	COMMENTS	COMPATIBILITY
500micrograms/1ml, 2.5mg/5ml for infusion	for broncho-dilation.	2.5mg/5ml ampoule or 5ml (2.5mg) with 500ml N/S, G or G/S to give a concentration of 3microgram/1ml or 5microgram/1ml.	5micrograms/ minute for 8-10 hours.	Monitor blood pressure, heart rate and blood glucose in diabetic patients. Pain at injection site may occur with S/C administration. Maternal pulmonary oedema, monitor hydration status of patient. Extravasation may cause tissue damage; for management guidelines see section A 7.	
	(C) IV infusion for pre-term labour via syringe pump.	Dilute 10ml (5mg) of the 2.5mg/5ml ampoule with G 40ml to produce a 100micrograms/1ml solution.	See package insert.	pH: 3-5 Flush: N/S or G. Sodium content: 0.15mmol/1ml. Other comments	
	(C) IV infusion for pre-term labour via volumetric infusion pump.	Dilute 10ml (5mg of the 2.5mg/5ml ampoule) with G 490ml to produce a 10micrograms/1ml solution.	See package insert.	IM and S/C injections are preferred to IV bolus for bronchodilation.	
	IM or S/C.	Ready diluted.			
	(C) S/C infusion via syringe pump for brittle asthmatics (unlicensed).	Ready diluted.	See specialist guidelines for details.		
Tetracosactrin Ampoule	IV bolus.	Ready diluted.	2 minutes.	**Acute Events Which May Accompany Administration** Hypersensitivity reactions, anaphylactic shock in patients with allergic disorders.	

DRUG AND FORMULATION	METHOD	INSTRUCTION FOR DILUTION AND SUITABLE DILUENT	ADMINISTER OVER	COMMENTS	COMPATIBILITY
250microgram/1ml				Extravasation may cause tissue damage; for management guidelines see section A 7. **pH:** 3.8-4.5 **Flush:** N/S.	
	IM.	Ready diluted.		**Sodium content:** negligible.	
Tetracycline Vial 250mg, 500mg	(I) IV infusion. See 'Other comments'.	Reconstitute 250mg vial with 5ml W and 500mg with 10ml W. Then dilute with at least 100ml (maximum 1 litre) N/S, G or G/S.	Minimum infusion time: 100ml over 5 minutes.	**Acute Events Which May Accompany Administration** Rapid infusion increases the risk of thrombophlebitis. Extravasation may cause tissue damage; for management guidelines see section A 7. **pH:** 1.8 **Flush:** N/S, G or G/S. **Sodium content:** nil. **Other comments** The use of a terminal in-line 0.2 micron filter is recommended by the manufacturer.	
Thiamine (unlicensed)	(I) IV infusion.	Dilute to 50-100ml with N/S.	10-30 minutes.	**Acute Events Which May Accompany Administration**	Do not administer with other drugs.

Notes

a) For abbreviations used in the table see section A 2.4

b) Prepare a fresh infusion every 24 hours unless otherwise specified.

DRUG AND FORMULATION	METHOD	INSTRUCTION FOR DILUTION AND SUITABLE DILUENT	ADMINISTER OVER	COMMENTS	COMPATIBILITY
Ampoule 100mg/1ml				Anaphylaxis. Sneezing and mild asthma are signs that further injections may cause lead to anaphylaxis. Extravasation may cause tissue damage; for management guidelines see section A 7. **pH:** 2.5-4.5 **Flush:** N/S. **Other comments**	
	IM.	Ready diluted.		Once diluted in N/S use within one hour.	
Thiopentone	IV bolus.	Reconstitute 500mg with 20ml W or 2.5g in 100ml W to produce a 2.5% solution. The dose may be further diluted with N/S or glucose (unlicensed diluent).	10-15 seconds.	**Acute Events Which May Accompany Administration** Hypotension, monitor blood pressure. Extravasation may cause tissue damage. Treat extravasation by immediate infiltration of hyaluronidase in a local anaesthetic. For general extravasation treatment guidelines see section A 7. **pH:** 10.5 (2.5% solution) **Flush:** N/S.	**Incompatible:** do not infuse with other drugs.
Ampoule 500mg Vial 2.5g	(I) IV infusion.	Reconstitute as above then dilute to 0.2-0.4% (2 to 4mg/1ml) with N/S or glucose (unlicensed diluent).		**Other comments** Check for haze or precipitation before administering. **Sodium content:** 4.9mmol/1g.	
	(C) IV infusion (unlicensed).	As for (I) IV infusion.			
Tobramycin	(I) IV infusion (preferred method).	Dilute required dose in 50-100ml N/S or G.	20-60 minutes.	**Acute Events Which May Accompany Administration** Allergic type reactions including anaphylaxis to the	**Y-site compatible (but see section A 2.6):** aciclovir (both drugs in glucose), ciprofloxacin,

DRUG AND FORMULATION	METHOD	INSTRUCTION FOR DILUTION AND SUITABLE DILUENT	ADMINISTER OVER	COMMENTS	COMPATIBILITY
Vial 20mg/2ml, 40mg/1ml, 80mg/2ml				preservative sodium bisulphite. Extravasation may cause tissue damage; for management guidelines see section A 7. **pH:** 3.5-6 **Flush:** N/S or G. **Other comments** Plasma level monitoring is required.	metronidazole. **Incompatible:** amoxycillin, azlocillin, cefotaxime, ceftazidime, cefuroxime, co-amoxiclav, flucloxacillin, heparin, teicoplanin, trimethoprim.
	IV bolus.	May be diluted with N/S or G.	3-5 minutes.		
	IM.	Ready diluted.			
Tramadol Ampoule 100mg/2ml	IV bolus.	Ready diluted.	2-3 minutes.	**Acute Events Which May Accompany Administration** Nausea, vomiting, skin rashes. Monitor for typical symptoms of opioid analgesic overdose. Treat with supportive measures and naloxone to reverse respiratory depression.	
	(I) or (C) IV infusion.	Dilute dose to a convenient volume in N/S, G or G/S.		**pH:** 6-6.8 **Flush:** N/S.	
	IM.	Ready diluted.		**Sodium content:** negligible.	
Tranexamic acid Ampoule	IV bolus (preferred method).	May be diluted with N/S or G.	100mg/minute.	**Acute Events Which May Accompany Administration** Rapid injection may cause dizziness and/or hypotension.	**Y-site compatible (but see section A 2.6):** heparin. **Incompatible:** penicillins.

Notes

a) For abbreviations used in the table see section A 2.4

b) Prepare a fresh infusion every 24 hours unless otherwise specified.

DRUG AND FORMULATION	METHOD	INSTRUCTION FOR DILUTION AND SUITABLE DILUENT	ADMINISTER OVER	COMMENTS	COMPATIBILITY
500mg/5ml	(C) IV infusion.	As above.	25-50mg/ kg/24 hours.	**pH:** 6.5-8 **Flush:** N/S or G. **Sodium content:** nil.	
TRH	See protirelin				
Trimetaphan Ampoule 250mg/5ml	(I) IV infusion (preferred method).	Dilute to 100-500ml with N/S or G/S to give a solution containing 500micrograms-2.5mg/1ml (usually 1mg/1ml).	Initially 3-4mg/ minute then adjust rate to produce required response.	**Acute Events Which May Accompany Administration** Monitor blood pressure as there is a marked variation in individual response. Tachycardia, monitor heart rate. **pH:** 5.2-5.5 **Flush:** N/S or G/S.	**Compatible in infusion bag (but see section A 2.6):** heparin. **Y-site compatible (but see section A 2.6):** potassium chloride. **Incompatible:** strongly alkaline agents e.g. thiopentone.
	IV bolus.	Ready diluted.		**Sodium content:** negligible.	
Trimethoprim Ampoule 100mg/5ml	IV bolus either directly or via a Y-site of a G drip.	May be diluted with G. "Monotrim" brand may be diluted with G, N/S or H if necessary.	Minimum 5 minutes.	**pH:** 4-4.5 **Flush:** G (Monotrim brand may be flushed with N/S). **Sodium content:** negligible.	**Incompatible:** aminoglycosides, metronidazole, sulphonamides. The "Syraprim" brand is incompatible with chloride ions.
Trimetrexate Vial 25mg	(I) IV infusion.	**Handle as for cytotoxic drugs.** Reconstitute each vial with 2ml of G or W. Dilute dose required in G to produce a	60-90 minutes.	**pH:** 3.5-5.5 (reconstituted in water) **Flush:** G or W. Do not flush with N/S. **Other comments** Cytotoxic drug, it should only be reconstituted in an	**Incompatible:** N/S, chloride ions, folinic acid.

DRUG AND FORMULATION	METHOD	INSTRUCTION FOR DILUTION AND SUITABLE DILUENT	ADMINISTER OVER	COMMENTS	COMPATIBILITY
		concentration of 0.25-2mg/1ml (e.g. 75mg in 100ml).		isolator by experienced staff. Trimetrexate must be given with folinic acid via a separate line.	
Urokinase Vial 5,000iu,	(I) IV infusion via syringe or volumetric	Reconstitute vial with 2-3ml W or N/S then further dilute with N/S to desired volume	Rate dependent on indication.	**Acute Events Which May Accompany Administration** Rapid administration may cause severe hypertension,	**Y-site compatible (but see section A 2.6):** heparin.

Notes

a) For abbreviations used in the table see section A 2.4

b) Prepare a fresh infusion every 24 hours unless otherwise specified.

DRUG AND FORMULATION	METHOD	INSTRUCTION FOR DILUTION AND SUITABLE DILUENT	ADMINISTER OVER	COMMENTS	COMPATIBILITY
25,000iu, 100,000iu	infusion pump.	which is dependent on indication.		cerebral haemorrhage and other bleeding. IV infusion should be administered where clinicians are experienced in thrombotic disease. If bleeding occurs stop infusion immediately and treat bleeding appropriately. **pH:** 5.5-7 **Flush:** N/S. **Sodium content:** negligible. **Other comments** Avoid IV in patients with active internal bleeding, cerebral embolism, CVA, aneurysm and uncontrolled hypertension.	
	IV bolus to unblock "AV" shunts and IV cannulae.	Reconstitute 5,000-25,000iu with 2-3ml N/S. To unblock haemodialysis lines, Permacaths, shunts and Hickman lines: leave to dwell in affected lumen for at least one hour and preferably 2-4 hours. Remove lysate and flush.			
acomycin g, 1g	(1) IV infusion.	Reconstitute each 500mg with 10ml W then dilute with a minimum of 100ml N/S or G. For fluid restricted patients see 'Other comments'.	Minimum 60 minutes. Doses over 500mg maximum rate	**Acute Events Which May Accompany Administration** Anaphylactoid reactions including hypotension, wheezing, dyspnoea, urticaria or pruritus. Rapid infusion may cause flushing of the upper body ('red	**Y-site compatible (but see section A 2.6):** aciclovir, fluconazole, morphine. **Incompatible:** amoxycillin, barbiturates, ceftazidime,

163

	INSTRUCTION FOR DILUTION AND SUITABLE DILUENT	ADMINISTER OVER	COMMENTS	COMPATIBILITY
		10mg/minute.	neck') or pain and muscle spasm of the chest and back. Extravasation may cause tissue damage; for management guidelines see section A 7. **pH:** 2.8-4.5 **Flush:** N/S or G. **Displacement:** 0.3ml/500mg vial. Add 9.7ml W to 500mg vial to give a concentration of 50mg/1ml. **Other comments** In practice 1g in 100ml is used in fluid restricted patients (unlicensed).	dexamethasone, fluconazole, foscarnet, heparin.
Vasopressin (synthetic)	See argipressin			
Vecuronium Vial 10mg	IV bolus Reconstitute with 5ml W (diluent provided). May be diluted to 1mg/1ml with W, N/S or G.	Rapidly.	**Acute Events Which May Accompany Administration** Erythematous reactions at injection site. **pH:** 4	**Y-site compatible (but see section A 2.6):** droperidol, fentanyl, midazolam, pancuronium, propofol, sodium nitroprusside. **Incompatible:** thiopentone and other alkaline agents.
	(C) IV infusion Reconstitute with 5ml W (diluent provided). Dilute with N/S or G to a maximum concentration of 4mg/100ml.		**Flush:** N/S or G.	
Verapamil Ampoule 5mg/2ml	IV bolus. May be diluted with N/S or G.	30 seconds.	**Acute Events Which May Accompany Administration** Reduced heart rate, transient hypotension, monitor blood pressure and **ECG.** Reduced contractility and in extreme cases asystole.	**Y-site compatible (but see section A 2.6):** digoxin.

Notes

a) For abbreviations used in the table see section A 2.4

b) Prepare a fresh infusion every 24 hours unless otherwise specified.

DRUG AND FORMULATION	METHOD	INSTRUCTION FOR DILUTION AND SUITABLE DILUENT	ADMINISTER OVER	COMMENTS	COMPATIBILITY
				Rarely flushing, headache, vertigo, allergic reactions. **pH:** 4-6.5 **Flush:** N/S. **Sodium content:** 0.3mmol/ampoule.	
Vigam-S	See Immunoglobulin human normal				
Vitamin B and C	See Pabrinex IVHP				
Vitamin K	See phytomenadione				
Zidovudine Vial 200mg/2ml	(C) IV infusion during labour (start infusion four hours before elective caesarean section).	Dilute to 2mg/1ml or 4mg/1ml with G. May be diluted with N/S if clinically indicated.	2mg/kg over 1 hour then 1mg/kg/hour until the umbilical cord is clamped.	**Acute Events Which May Accompany Administration** May cause pain, irritation and phlebitis at injection site. **pH:** 5.5 **Flush:** N/S or G. **Other comments** Discard unused infusion after 8 hours at room temperature.	**Y-site compatible (but see section A 2.6):** clindamycin (both drugs in G).